The Prepper's Long-Term Survival Handbook
&
Off Grid Living

2-in-1 Compilation

Step By Step Guide to Become Completely Self Sufficient and Survive Any Disaster in as Little as 30 Days

Small Footprint Press

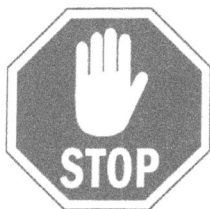

BEFORE YOU START READING, DOWNLOAD YOUR FREE BONUSES!

Scan the QR-code & Access
all the Resources for FREE!

SCAN ME

The Self-Sufficient Living Cheat Sheet

10 Simple Steps to Become More Self-Sufficient in 1 Hour or Less

How to restore balance to the environment around you... even if you live in a tiny apartment in the city.

Discover:

- **How to increase your income** by selling "useless" household items
- The environmentally friendly way to replace your car — invest in THIS special vehicle to **eliminate your carbon footprint**
- The secret ingredient to **turning your backyard into a thriving garden**
- 17+ different types of food scraps and 'waste' that you can use to feed your garden
- How to drastically **cut down on food waste** without eating less
- 4 natural products you can use to make your own eco-friendly cleaning supplies
- The simple alternative to 'consumerism' — the age-old method for **getting what you need without paying money for it**
- The 9 fundamental items you need to create a self-sufficient first-aid kit
- One of the top skills that most people are afraid of learning — and how you can master it effortlessly
- 3 essential tips for **gaining financial independence**

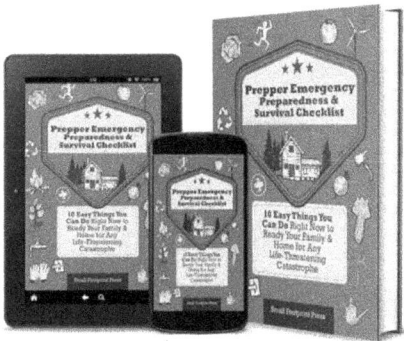

The Prepper Emergency Preparedness & Survival Checklist:

10 Easy Things You Can Do Right Now to Ready Your Family & Home for Any Life-Threatening Catastrophe

Natural disasters demolish everything in their path, but your peace of mind and sense of safety don't have to be among them. Here's what you need to know...

- Why having an emergency plan in place is so crucial and how it will help to keep your family safe

- How to stockpile emergency supplies intelligently and why you shouldn't overdo it

- How to store and conserve water so that you know you'll have enough to last you through the crisis

- A powerful 3-step guide to ensuring financial preparedness, no matter what happens

- A step-by-step guide to maximizing your storage space, so you and your family can have exactly what you need ready and available at all times

- Why knowing the hazards of your home ahead of time could save a life and how to steer clear of these in case of an emergency

- Everything you need to know for creating a successful evacuation plan, should the worst happen and you need to flee safely

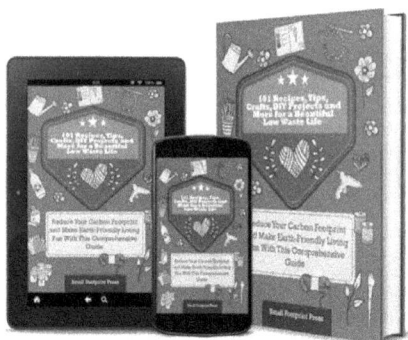

101 Recipes, Tips, Crafts, DIY Projects and More for a Beautiful Low Waste Life

Reduce Your Carbon Footprint and Make Earth-Friendly Living Fun With This Comprehensive Guide

Practical, easy ways to improve your personal health and habits while contributing to a brighter future for yourself and the planet

Discover:

- **Simple customizable recipes for creating your own food, home garden, and skincare products**

- The tools you need for each project to successfully achieve sustainable living

- Step-by-step instructions for life-enhancing skills from preserving food to raising your own animals and forging for wild berries

- **Realistic life changes that reduce your carbon-footprint while saving you money**

- Sustainable crafts that don't require any previous knowledge or expertise

- Self-care that extends beyond the individual and positively impacts the environment

- **Essential tips on how to take back control of your life -- become self-sustained and independent**

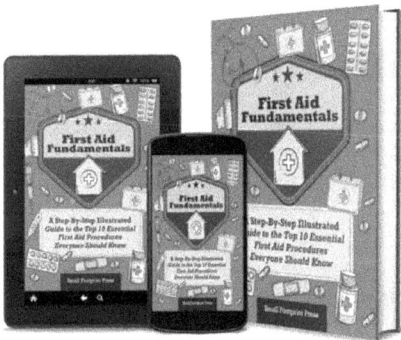

First Aid Fundamentals

A Step-By-Step Illustrated Guide to the Top 10 Essential First Aid Procedures Everyone Should Know

Discover:

- **What you should do to keep this type of animal attack from turning into a fatal allergic reaction**
- Why sprains are more than just minor injuries, and how you can keep them from getting worse
- **How to make the best use of your environment in critical situations**
- The difference between second- and third-degree burns, and what you should do when either one happens
- Why treating a burn with ice can actually cause more damage to your skin
- When to use heat to treat an injury, and when you should use something cold
- **How to determine the severity of frostbite**, and what you should do in specific cases
- Why knowing this popular disco song could help you save a life
- The key first aid skill that everyone should know — **make sure you learn THIS technique the right way**

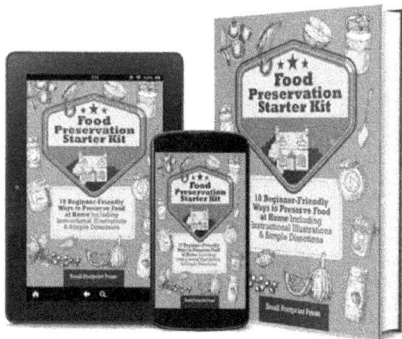

Food Preservation Starter Kit

10 Beginner-Friendly Ways to Preserve Food at Home | Including Instructional Illustrations and Simple Directions

Grocery store prices are skyrocketing! It's time for a self-sustaining lifestyle.

Discover:

- **10 incredibly effective and easy ways to preserve your food for a self-sustaining lifestyle**

- The art of canning and the many different ways you can preserve food efficiently without any prior experience

- A glorious trip down memory lane to learn the historical methods of preservation passed down from one generation to the next

- **How to make your own pickled goods**: enjoy the tanginess straight from your kitchen

- Detailed illustrations and directions so you won't feel lost in the preservation process

- The health benefits of dehydrating your food and how fermentation can be **the key to a self-sufficient life**

- **The secrets to living a processed-free life** and saving Mother Earth all at the same time

Download all your resources by scanning the QR-Code below:

Table of Contents

The Prepper's Long-Term Survival Handbook

Off-Grid Living

The Prepper's Long-Term Survival Handbook

2-in-1 Compilation

Step By Step Guide to Become Completely Self Sufficient and Survive Any Disaster in as Little as 30 Days

Small Footprint Press

Introduction

Our society is becoming increasingly unstable—our world functions in more unsustainable ways with each passing day. With the planet's growing population, an affinity for a faster-paced life, advancements in technology, and a preference for an increasingly self-centered lifestyle for many individuals, our environmental resources are being depleted faster than we can imagine. Our current situation shows that in the future, we may have to seek alternative ways to live. Let's imagine that the unthinkable happens, and say a global market crash, a world-altering natural disaster, famine, or large-scale war occurs. At that moment, we'll realize that the need to be prepared for such things is absolutely crucial. But it's no use waiting for these kinds of disasters to take place. It's time to act now. But you may ask, where do I even start? The answer is simple: educate yourself on what to prepare for, the ways you can prep, and how. After learning more about it, you can then take the practical steps to build a framework to create your plan of action. The prepping lifestyle isn't just about stocking piles of food and water. It starts with changing your mindset that foresees events before they take place and taking the proper action to mitigate the effects of these events. There is a common notion among non-preppers that preppers are paranoid kinds of people. But nothing could be further from the truth! Preppers are simply individuals that have developed a mentality to plan for the future, take the initiative in taking care of themselves and their families, and utilize their resources in the most efficient way.

One example that shows how important it is to be prepared is a recent event that we have all experienced. At the beginning of 2020, the world was hit by the Covid-19 pandemic. Because of the announcement of a lockdown, people panicked and flocked to stores to try and stock up on food and other supplies. Mass shortages occurred, and people were then faced with the fear of a virus *and* running out of food. This short-sighted approach to dealing with a crisis was the least efficient way to deal with the situation, and consequences took forth. For preppers who had been prepared to deal with this, panicking and running out to buy things wasn't so necessary. Preparing in advance allows less disruption when crises come. These kinds of events truly make us realize the need to prep.

We understand that prepping can be an arduous activity and that the thought of going off the grid can be an uncertain and complex task. The very notion of leaving everything behind scares people because they have no idea at first what to expect. In a society dependent on the government to care for the people's every need, many might doubt if they would be able to survive at all without being closely linked to government-provided services. We also understand that you, the reader, may still be a beginner and think that you don't have the necessary skills to be able to survive in wilderness situations and that the thought of such cases can sound frightening. Or maybe you're a camping or survivalist enthusiast, and you want to leap at the chance of becoming more independent and getting out of the stress of the city. Whatever your station in life is, this book aims to provide the answers for you. This book is the perfect resource for anyone thinking of tackling the great outdoors. You'll learn about the first steps to living off the grid so that you can set up a sustainable off-grid home. You'll also receive tips and advice on how to protect yourself and your family in survival situations. Finally, if you're an experienced outdoor lover, you'll learn how to survive and thrive in nature, the place you treasure the most. Whatever problem you may be facing, this book aims to teach you one key skill: preparedness.

Other outdoor guides can seem confusing and restricted to only those with no experience having the right equipment, knowledge, or skills. These guides may not be as helpful to someone just starting to get into the prepper movement. Many guides seem to only focus on the countryside or wilderness survival. Fewer of them seem to deal with the need to survive in the urban environment, which is just as important because many emergencies can happen even if you're not outdoors. Prepping is for all times and all seasons. This guide aims to give you a truly holistic view of the topic of prepping. We won't assume that you're an expert in this sort of thing, and we'll start with the beginning by laying out the foundational concepts and give a plan of action. We also won't assume that you have access to expensive forms of equipment, so we'll show you how you can make use of the most basic of tools to live in an efficient and environmentally friendly way.

So, what kind of topics does this book cover? First, we'll give you the facts on the most crucial survival skills, what these survival abilities mean, how to learn these skills, and which real-life situations in which these skills can be best used. Then, we'll guide you to using these same skills in an urban environment and in the wilderness. Each step-by-step plan will be presented in an easy-to-read and practical fashion. Next, we'll explain to you all of the possible situations that you might need to prep for and how best to employ the skills learned in this book in such cases. This book covers the basics of survival 101, how to find water in hostile environments, finding food, and how to stay warm during the night in frigid conditions. We'll also discuss how to administer first aid, take care of yourself in the city and the wild. Lastly, we'll also help guide you in building shelters for various kinds of environments and using different kinds of tools and materials. However, the most important skill that this book will teach is how to develop the mindset of a survivor. What you do when you find yourself in perilous situations is important, but the mentality that you'll need for it is the backbone for all your plans. Preparing yourself mentally is possibly the most vital skill you can master in this life. It will see you through many scrapes and pitfalls. Developing a can-do attitude allows you to take the initiative and control situations rather than be controlled by them.

Who is Small Footprint Press?

"Accelerating Sustainable Survival for the Individual and our Planet"

"Prepping to survive a global catastrophe goes hand-in-hand with stopping the destruction of our planet by living sustainably!" Small Footprint Press Company Values.

While we aren't doomers who focus solely on disasters and collapses or on beliefs that the end of the world is nearing, we do believe in being prepared for the worst while living your best life each day. For this reason, we work toward promoting and encouraging sustainable, prepared living as an individual. While we guide individuals on prepping, we also teach the importance of living sustainably and self-sufficiently. Did you know that in 2021 over 45 percent of Americans, both men, and women, are investing in prepping for worst-case scenarios? (Laycock & Choi, 2021) We're not just talking about stockpiling food and toilet paper, but also equipment and taking instructional courses. It is only by realizing the fragility of the planet we inhabit that we can begin to develop the right attitude towards it. The future of the world as we know it is in our hands. We have to take steps to be prepared for any and every eventuality, and this book is the perfect starting point for that. The knowledge in this book is not intended solely as a guide for when you find yourself in those situations, but more a guide to being prepared for the situations you might find yourself in in the future.

Who is this book for?

This book is for men and women of all ages who want to have a hand in the destiny of our planet. It is for individuals concerned with the current state of the environment and who seek to make a tangible difference in their lives and the futures of everyone who lives on planet earth. Those who desire self-sufficiency and freedom from the government will love this book because it teaches the skills needed in order to be independent. Those from all walks of life are welcome to take the "independence challenge" and free themselves from the restrictions of modern life. Throughout your journey, this book will be your constant companion.

Chapter 1:
The Basics of Survival

In light of the current world situation politically, economically, and in every other way, it is vital to have an understanding of the basics surrounding survival techniques. When difficult situations arise, as they often do, only those who are prepared will be able to not only survive but thrive in such situations. In order to build a framework for survival knowledge, you need to be able to educate yourself on the basic techniques first. To understand why wilderness survival is so important, you first have to understand the world you live in and the environment that is around you. Understanding the basics of survival is the first step to becoming truly independent in every area of your life and not have to rely entirely on governmental forces and establishments. So, while many think of prepping as being all doom and gloom, the opposite remains true. It is a chance to truly experience independence and finally enjoy present life, being prepared for the worst-case scenarios.

Why does Wilderness Survival Matter?

In the comfortable urban environment that many people find themselves in, survival is not a priority because they have access to everything they need when they need it. There is no need to take unnecessary risks to obtain rewards, in other words. Society has conditioned people into not having to fight for what they want. They are far too reliant on the government. However, unless we're planning on not living on Earth in the next few years, it would seem like a wise idea to learn these basic survival techniques. Before the advent of technology, humans always knew how to survive on what they had and often made do with little in the way of resources. These days, this is no longer a consideration. But life is unpredictable. The best way to safeguard ourselves and our loved ones for the future is by developing our skills in the area of survival and encouraging those we know and love to do the same.

A crucial reason why survival skills matter is because of the constant change of our climate. Climate change is a latent threat that cannot be ignored for much longer. When the crises caused by this climate change come, our response will be proportionate to how much we've prepared for these moments. In order to combat the devastating situations caused by climate change, it would be wise to create a climate change response plan. This climate change action could be part of a much larger movement towards disconnecting from harmful practices that affect the environment. Think of it as a way to free yourself from the constraints of being connected to the grid so you can explore a new life. This book offers hope from the doom and gloom of the constant news we see each day. With the right mindset and plan, you can find freedom in being self-sufficient and ready.

How Does the World Respond to the Danger of Climate Change?

The globe is vast, and there are many cities in it. Each of these cities produces carbon emissions that affect the climate in some way, to a greater or lesser degree. A large number of people live in these coastal cities. Due to the rising sea levels, large numbers of these people will have to relocate, and the only way they can go is inland. However, there may be many more ways that people displaced can live. Newer innovations such as environmentally restorative communities are being created, even as we speak. These communities are being considered possible living spaces in the future by those who inhabit smaller islands because their homes may cease to exist in the future. These communities consist of a bunch of interconnected houses on floating platforms connected by small bridges and which contain gardens. On top of each roof is a green roof, or a type of vegetation positioned over a layer of waterproofing. But, how does all of this tie into the idea of creating a climate change disaster plan? The notion that there are innovations being thought of points towards the fact that there are climate change disaster plans being formulated. This planning can be applied to the individual. What can we do to develop sustainable plans for the future in our own lives and families?

As a start, it's important to know that there are different kinds of survivalists. Some are the typical preppers you sometimes see portrayed in the media as the gun-hoarding, food-stockpiling, disaster-predicting type. Next, there are those who take the job a little more seriously. Those who are farmers are technologically advanced and have methods of survival, which include open-source plans for every single kind of machinery and equipment that they need. Finally, there are those who have a simpler mentality: they believe that survival is just about survival and are quite happy to make use of as little or as much as they need in order to get by. What kind of plan you want to create depends on what your goals are. If you just want to live in a more environmentally friendly way, there are many ways to start planning to do this. The first thing you need to understand is how to survive in the wilderness. This involves a fundamental grasp of what bushcraft means. There is a real difference between what bushcraft means and what survival skills mean. Survival methods, or skills, refer to the ways in which you deal with difficult and unexpected emergencies when you are forced to fend for yourself. The goal in any survival situation is to make your way to safety. Bushcraft is an often voluntary exercise that requires you to make use of nature to sustain yourself for long periods. For example, someone practicing bushcraft might take a long period of time out in the woods and live on nothing but the land. On the other hand, someone who is in a survival situation might have been dropped there in a plane crash and have no means of immediate escape from the situation. The difference between survival skills and bushcraft are the types of situations and the urgency of these situations to a large degree. Let us examine bushcraft in more detail.

What is Bushcraft?

There are three main things you cannot survive without, no matter where you may find yourself. These things are well-known: water, food, and shelter. If you take two or even just one of these things away, your chance of survival drops from poor to none at all. Fortunately, there are courses that you can take that can help you to gain the skills you need to be more prepared in case you ever end up in a situation without the most basic necessities. Engaging in bushcraft activities is a great way to ensure that you get the type of mental and physical preparation you need in order to prepare for the most extreme of situations. Bushcraft mainly deals with the techniques you need to survive, but what if you are intending on spending a longer period of time in the wilderness? You'll need to pick up other skills that will help you to grow beyond just the three basic needs. These skills can also be incorporated into the term "learning bushcraft," This is also where bushcraft and survival skills tend to diverge. Survival skills are a lot more restrictive in terms of the fact that they are limited to a specific set of circumstances. On the other hand, bushcraft tends to think of the more long-term practicalities of being in the wilderness, and the amount of things that need to be learned is much greater as a result. There is a greater urgency with survival skills. There are necessities that cannot be ignored. With bushcraft, the pace of the whole experience is slower and can be seen as a learning experience rather than a life and death struggle. There are, however, specific skills that are common to both kinds of experiences. Let us look at some of these skills. They may vary in significance depending on the urgency of the situation and the context surrounding the person engaging in these skills and activities.

Tools

In order to survive in the wild, you'll need to learn how to use specific tools. These tools can give you access to the resources you need to not only survive but live comfortably. Some tools are limited in their use and are therefore only useful for extreme survival situations. Other tools are not as vital but are useful and helpful to have in order to make living easier. Whatever your needs may be, you'll need to be able to use the tools that you have at your disposal and sometimes even make your own in order to survive. In addition, learning to use tools will make you more independent.

Fire

The second skill you'll need to possess is the ability to make fire. Fire is unquestionably one of the most significant challenges that many survivalists face in extreme situations. You need to be aware of the different methods to create a fire depending on where you are and the tools that are available to you. The challenge in creating fire is not just in having the proper materials, but in that, you also need the right skills to be able to get it started. The climate and the wood's condition also have to be suitable to get a fire going. These things might not necessarily be in your control, so a lot of what you need requires the circumstances to be in your favor. You can, however, control how you use these circumstances to your advantage. Skills you'll need when building a fire include the following:

- Finding and stacking tinder

- Collecting and preparing wood

- Building a fire-making tool

- Building a fire pit

- Making and utilizing different kinds of fire for specific purposes

Not all fire is used as a heating device. Sometimes, it is constructed for other purposes. You will need to be aware of what these purposes are and how to best make use of them when the situation arises.

Shelter

Constructing a shelter takes knowledge of what materials to use and how to put these materials together in a way that makes a place where you can stay warm and dry and protected from the elements and dangers. It is vital to have skills in shelter building because without them, you could perish from the bad weather or freezing temperatures in a matter of hours. Here are the skills you'll need in order to build a shelter include the following: knowledge of woodcraft and woodworking skills, harvesting other materials, thatch weaving, making knots, making waterproofing, and more. For cold climates where there is actual ice and snow, you'll need to be able to make use of the snow to create your shelter, which requires a set of skills and knowledge all on its own. Depending on the situation you find yourself in, you'll have to learn to construct shelters of varying degrees of complexity. In an off-grid situation, you'll need to plan before you can build a shelter.

Water

Without water, you will perish. This is an absolute certainty, and thus the need for water takes precedence over everything else. When you find yourself in a difficult situation, you need to stop and think about where you can find vital resources. Knowledge of where to begin and how you're going to exploit these resources are critical to being prepared. What will you do if the traditional sources of water such as springs, lakes, and rivers aren't available? How will you purify water once you've found it? What will you do to make it drinkable? Such skills can only come through educating yourself. The skills you'll need include the following: water identification, water purification skills, making filters, building a fire, and creating containers for storing your water.

Food

Food is secondary when it comes to water, but it is still critical for you to find. Without food, you could perish in a few days. Food gives you the energy to keep moving. Without it, in any survival situation, you could easily fade out and die. Knowing where to find food and what is edible is not always common knowledge. People in survival situations know they have to eat, but they often lack the knowledge of what plants are safe to ingest and what animals are fit for consumption. For example, you may want to fish for food, but do you know the best way to do this? Where are the best places to fish in the river, for example? Is fishing done only with a line and reel, or are there other ways? This guide aims to help you discover more about how you can gather, safely prepare, and eat in all kinds of extreme situations. These are skills you'll need to be able to find food: foraging, hunting skills, the ability to fish and to create traps that can catch fish, the ability to capture small animals to eat, cleaning and cooking game, tracking game, and using scent concealers, use of different weapons to trap prey, and many more.

Navigation

If you're in an emergency situation and you want to find your way out of it, you'll need to be absolutely adept with your navigational skills. Finding your way from point A to point B isn't as simple as walking there. There are obstacles to overcome, and you definitely need to be sure you're heading the right way. The wilderness, combined with the shock and trauma of being lost, can be a disorienting place. You need to be mentally, physically, and emotionally prepared to plan ahead and figure out how you are going to get to safety. Your very life could depend on your ability to navigate using the tools you have. These tools aren't only the compass you have in your bag. Sometimes, you might have to rely on the sun and the stars to lead you. Having this knowledge tucked away can be a literal lifesaver.

First Aid

First aid is not only about applying quick and effective remedies to others; you also need it to save your own life. First aid is an absolutely necessary and critical skill. If you're wounded and lost, you'll need to first ensure that you remain alive so that you can access the resources you need in order to start planning your escape. Your good health is paramount at this point. And taking care of that health starts with being aware of first aid. Skills you'll need to be able to administer first aid, either to yourself or to others: the ability to do CPR, splint or stitch wounds, apply bandages, stop bleeding, make use of various kinds of plants and natural materials to attend to the sick, and many other skills.

All of these skills and more will be covered in further depth through future chapters. However, the main thing to realize is that this book is here to help layout all the things you need to gain your independence.

Survival Gear Checklist

Before you start your survival journey, you'll need to make sure you've got everything you need. The items on this list are primarily aimed at people who are interested in taking up bushcraft, but they can be applied in extreme emergency situations as well. If you know what items to use in these situations, you can make use of similar items when you find yourself in an emergency. Lack of preparedness can never be an excuse when faced with tough situations. Always prepare accordingly, and you'll put yourself in the best position to survive. The items on this list are divided into the different categories you're going to require them to be used. Sometimes, items will fit into more than one category. While you may not be able to carry everything on this list, you can try and approximate what you need based on the situation that you may find yourself in. You can begin to gather these materials months in advance if you're planning a trip. It is always good to have a kit that you can keep adding to before and when the situation demands it. It's important to realize that your *gear* can be collected in advance, but supplies will need to be gathered when necessary, as some things may not last. Always do your research on what you need. Always keep a kit available in your car and one in your home for emergencies.

Water filtration and purification items

To purify water and make it safe to drink, you'll require a mini water filter and water purification tablets. Together, these items can save you a nasty case of dysentery or an even worse water-borne illness while you're in the wilderness. Always be sure to take a water bottle with you. These can be used to store and water as you travel. A water bottle will be able to keep you hydrated while you're moving between sources of water. Make sure your bottle is made of metal so that it can be heated if you need to boil your water. In a world that is becoming increasingly water-scarce, proper conservation and treatment of water are also vital.

Shelters

Building your own shelter is a huge and critical step of the survival process. In order to create a livable shelter, you'll require a survival tarp or a piece of material that you can use as a cover. You can also invest in a tent that is easy to carry from place to place, and that can be easily installed. The disadvantage of a tent is that it can be heavy to carry, but it can serve you very well once it is set up. Hammocks are great if you're traveling in finer weather. They can also work in inclement weather and keep your body off the ground, something other sleeping arrangements might not be able to do. A hammock tent provides both the comfort of a hammock and the shelter of a survival tarp. These will tend to be more expensive. When all else fails, you can invest in a sleeping bag and an emergency blanket. These are relatively inexpensive and can be used in a pinch. Always be aware of the type of weather you might encounter before you start your survival journey and invest accordingly. Your shelter will depend on the type of climate you're in.

Weapons

When referring to weapons in a survival context, these are the things that you will need to use in the chance that you end up in a situation where you'll need to defend yourself. You would also be needing weapons that you can use to be able to hunt and fish. Finally, you're going to need weapons to use as tools, such as saws and axes. Let us look a little more closely at the types of tools you're going to need.

The first thing on your list is going to be a firearm, which is a sophisticated kind of weapon even at the best of times and requires some investment and expertise. If you're already trained, a firearm will be at the top of your list. Note that the ammo is considered survival supplies. There is no one size fits all approach to owning a firearm. However, when you're embarking on a survival mission, you'll want to choose the one that is light and efficient, as well as a weapon that is most reliable. You also need to make sure you have enough ammo to protect yourself, your family and to use for other tasks. If you're intending on hunting with your weapon, ensure that it is a weapon that has the ability to take down the caliber of prey that you want. Some kinds of weapons can be used for both self-defense and for hunting. Be sure to do your research before acquiring the type of weapon you want and also acquire the licenses that you might need. Bear in mind that you may or may not be able to simply discharge firearms at will. Be aware of the environments you find yourself in at all times.

Invest in a snake bore. A snake bore is a bore cleaner that is a must for anyone owning a firearm. Proper maintenance of your weapon is essential when you're in the wilderness. You'll need everything to function as it should.

You could also make your own weapons to use in the

field. You can design and build these weapons as and when you need them while you're in the wilderness, but you may not have the materials and equipment you need. A better idea is to design what you need beforehand. Such customizable weapons include homemade knives, stun guns, and flamethrowers.

A bow and arrow is another essential item if you're planning on hunting. These weapons are perfect when stealth is required, and a firearm simply will not work. Their disadvantage is that they require some level of proficiency in order to operate properly, and conditions have to be optimal for their most effective use. Crossbows also fit into this category.

A tactical pen is also a weapon you might want to keep on your person. These are hardened metal pens with ink cartridges inside that are under pressure. They do not kill but can still be used to strike an opponent as a last resort. In addition, they are, of course, pens and can be used for making notes, maps, and many more helpful purposes.

Stun guns are useful for discharging a blast of electricity that will leave an opponent indisposed for a few moments. They are useful for self-defense only and are not 100% reliable. However, when they do work, they are perfect for situations where you're faced with imminent danger.

Mace spray is a substance that comes in small pressurized containers. It can be discharged at the faces of potential predators and enemies. It has a range of up to 20 feet.

In addition to these weapons, there are the usual spears, knives, machetes, saws, and other kinds of similar weapons you'll be needing to carry out tasks while you're on the trail.

Fire Starting Kit

Fire starting is synonymous with survival in the wilderness. Your ability to get a fire started could be the difference between life and death. It's not enough to simply learn to start a fire. You'll need to be able to adapt to the conditions you'll find yourself in quickly. Bear in mind that sometimes you're going to need to start a fire in a downpour or when it's sleeting or snowing. How will you preserve the integrity of your fire-making materials? Where will you find dry tinder or wood? Such knowledge has to be obtained before heading out on the trail. You'll need a lighter that works in all kinds of weather conditions. It is worth investing in a good one.

You could also invest in a ferro rod. This is a small device that requires no gas and is good for nearly 12,000 uses. It is also extremely reliable for creating a spark. They require a small amount of practice to use but are otherwise an extremely valuable addition to your survival kit.

Matches are useful to have around, but they are susceptible to getting wet in difficult conditions and can be rendered useless. However, you can purchase the waterproof variety that has some degree of durability in unfavorable conditions.

You can purchase something known as fire laces. These are shoelace-like items that have ferro rods attached to the end of them. These are easy to carry because you can thread them into your shoes, and you'll always have access to fire-making materials no matter where you are.

If you really want to start a fire, however, you're going to be relying heavily on a tinder box. Having access to dry tinder will always help you start a fire, no matter the conditions you find yourself in. In addition, some tinderboxes have built-in graters that you can use to break down dry wood so that it is easily usable as tinder.

Bladed Tools

A survival shovel is a tool used for displacing dirt, digging holes and trenches, and clearing the ground so that you can establish a campsite. It is a versatile and necessary tool and will perform tasks that you cannot do with a knife, for example.

A survival knife is a fixed-bladed implement that you will need to cut through stubborn items. It is an essential part of your survival kit. Be sure to invest in a knife that is durable and weatherproof.

An axe is a versatile tool that can be used for cutting down trees, cutting through branches, and for self-defense purposes. In a pinch, they can be used for hunting. Survival hatchets are another kind of survival axe but smaller.

A multitool is a device that has many different functions. Some are shaped like knives and have pliers attached to them. These pliers are very useful when you're in a situation where you need to remove objects or items that you can't grip with your fingers. These tools also have other bladed tools attached to them, like bottle openers, corkscrews, and other small bladed implements.

A multipurpose credit card tool is a tool shaped like a credit card that can be opened to reveal various useful items, such as knives and picks. These don't typically come with a set of pliers attached, but they are lightweight and versatile nonetheless.

Blade sharpeners are a must if you're planning on spending an extended amount of time in the wilderness. Your knives are your most important tools. They need to be cared for, and learning how to sharpen a knife and actually sharpening it are necessary skills. If your blade is blunt and unable to perform the purpose of which it is intended, it can put you at risk. Always take care of your tools.

Rescue Items

When you're in the wilderness, and you're seeking rescue, you need to have specific tools that will help you attract attention and possibly save your life. Unfortunately, in many instances, you will eventually have to improvise in your use of these tools.

Whistle

A signal whistle makes a sound that can be heard from a long way off, and it can draw attention to your plight. If someone is in the area, they might not be able to see your signal, but they could possibly hear it if it is loud enough.

Signal Mirror

A signal mirror is a mirror used to reflect the light of the sun onto specific objects. These are effective at being seen from many miles away.

Colorful items

If you don't have these items, you can improvise by creating a fire or by using colorful items, such as brightly colored clothing to attract attention. Discarded parachutes, for example, are often brightly colored and can be used to create eye-catching signals in a pinch. Always make sure that you keep fabrics and materials around with you if you find yourself in a survival situation.

Miscellaneous Survival Items

There are numerous other items that might be essential to your survival but are often overlooked. Depending on where you are, you might want to invest in fishing tackle. It is useful when you're attempting to fish and can be easily stored. You'll also want to have a flashlight on you. Tactical flashlights don't need batteries to be charged and can be priceless in a difficult situation, particularly if you're struggling to make a fire. Finally, consider investing in a survival pack in which you can keep all your smaller items. Other larger items can be carried on a tactical belt if you have one.

Survival Mentality

What is meant by a survival mentality? A survival mentality is the mindset of a winner in every situation that you find yourself in. It is the most important weapon in your arsenal, and in some situations, it could be the difference between life and death. So, why is a winner's mentality so important when you find yourself in a struggle for survival?

Planning and Preparation

First of all, a survival mentality helps you to remain positive in all circumstances. With this positivity comes confidence that you can carry out the tasks that you need to and that you can take the necessary steps in order to survive. Positivity breeds confidence, and confidence breeds success. In a life or death struggle, you need all the positivity you can get. If you have already cultivated this mindset, you're already on your way to coming out on top in any survival situation. You may not be able to predict the future, but you can always be mentally ready for it.

A strong mentality is one of self-reliance. The ability to do things for yourself and to be able to adapt to different situations is the mentality that you will need in many difficult situations. There are practical steps that you can take to make sure that you are able to cope with whatever comes your way. The ability to be self-reliant comes from a quality that is inherent in all of us, but only some make use of it. It is the ability to plan and organize for the future. Proper planning is a sign that you have the mentality of a winner because you're able to put into practice the ideas that you have, you know that these ideas will work, and you're able to organize them in a coherent way.

Planning sometimes requires sacrifice, but those with a strong desire to win will be willing to put everything on the line in order to achieve their goals. The mentality of a winner doesn't only apply to survival situations. You need to have a never-say-die attitude in every aspect of life. You never know when you will require it.

Dealing With Anxiety

When you're out on the trail, there are times when you will start to feel overwhelmed by situations that you never thought you would encounter, no matter what your skill level in survivalism may be. We all get scared. This is a fact of life. But some people never appear to be rushed or concerned in any way. Why is this? It is because, a long time ago, they learned that whenever they're faced with a situation that threatens to derail their confidence, you have to remain outwardly and inwardly calm. This inner peace enables them to not panic in situations.

For the vast majority of us, though, fear is something that we don't generally tend to handle very well, like that the massive spider in the bathroom that causes us to lose our cool or a large, frightening, and noisy dog for some people. These are relatively minor disturbances. But when we're lost in the jungle, the threat is suddenly made more real in a disorienting and claustrophobic environment.

Death can often occur in a matter of hours unless you're able to keep it together and take the necessary steps to extricate yourself from the predicament. So, how do we overcome fear in simple terms?

The first step is to identify the source of the anxiety. What is causing you to lose your mental focus at that moment? Let's take one hypothetical example: you're lost, there's a predator near you in the forest, and you know it's a wolf (even if you can't see it). Once you've identified that it is a wolf, the next step is to determine whether the fear is a rational or irrational fear. In the case of a wolf, the fear is most certainly rational and, therefore, a security feature in your mind. It stops you from going near that wolf instead of leading you into a panic. With the knowledge you now have, you're able to make a detour around the area where the wolf is, and you can avoid the danger. This is how fear works. We need to harness it to make ourselves stronger.

Our bodies are a cocktail of different chemicals, and when someone is stressed, certain hormones are pumped into the body. When we're in the grip of these hormones, they can affect how we react to situations. If we react negatively, we could end up making a situation that endangers ourselves or others. The key is to harness this fear and use it to our advantage.

The next step is to latch onto something bigger than ourselves. What drives us to succeed? What are some times when we've faced similar situations and overcome them? What are some times when we've faced situations and gotten through them, even though we didn't think we could? Latch onto these former times and remind yourself of what you're capable of and who you truly are. Then, you can do what you set your mind to. Activate your faith, whatever that may be to you. Remember a loved one. Harness the power of your emotions to take control of yourself, and thus your situation.

Survival Mindset Traits

There are certain traits within someone that's a survivor compared to a person who is not. In fact, we can all survive if we choose to change our attitudes towards life and towards our circumstances. Tenacity, adaptability, work ethic, creativity, positivity, acceptance, humor, bravery, and motivation are some of the qualities you need in order to effectively cope with the situations you find yourself in on a day-to-day basis. Let's look at a few of these traits.

Tenacity

Tenacity is the ability to remain steadfast even in the midst of difficulty. Tenacity has nothing to do with your physical fortitude or even your state of mind sometimes. It is a manifestation of your will to overcome any and every situation. Tenacity is fighting against your own desire to give up, even when this would seem easier than carrying on. However, tenacity alone is hard to maintain when the struggles of life are constantly beating you down. Guilt, fatigue, stress, anxiety, fear, and worry can all gnaw away at your inner strength. You have to maintain this inner strength throughout your ordeal. Talking to others can help if you're in a position where you're stranded with others. If you're on your own, this is more difficult. Invent distractions as a way of keeping your mind busy.

Adaptability

Adaptability is the ability to evolve according to changing situations and seasons and change the way you think and feel. In survival terms, this means, for example, that you won't act the same way in a forest as you will in a jungle. They are different environments and require different ways of operating. Having the knowledge and skills to be able to function in every kind of climate, weather, situation, or biome is known as being adaptable. Obstacles to your adaptability can be stubbornness and resistance to change. The way you can overcome this is by opening up your mind to different possibilities and solutions.

Work Ethic

Work ethic is a mental quality as well as a physical one. The desire to work hard starts in your mind. Survival is about hard work. In order to keep yourself alive, you have to work hard at performing the tasks that you need to perform. The downside is that you can often be hindered in your desire to work by things like circumstance, bodily injury, and factors beyond your control. Sometimes, there is nothing else to do in such situations, but to the best you can until circumstances are more favorable again. You may want to build a sophisticated and warm shelter, but it might be raining and impossible to do anything. The only option left to you might be to hide in a cave and wait out the rain. Such is the need for adaptability when you cannot perform the work that you really want to do.

Creativity

Creativity is a quality that allows you to think outside of the box. Hindrances to creativity might be fear of getting something wrong if you take a step outside the box. The way to overcome this is to get over your fear of failure. When you're in a life or death situation, you need to think of new ways to overcome difficult situations.

Positivity

Positivity is an overlooked quality when you're in a tense struggle for survival. All your effort might be so focused on getting through the experience that you forget to be thankful for what you already have. When you have a positive and determined attitude, difficult situations seem easier.

Acceptance

Acceptance of circumstances doesn't mean you accept their difficulties as well. It means that you acknowledge where you are at and are willing to make the necessary changes to get out of the situation.

Humor

Humor isn't just for clowns. Humor in difficult situations

can actually be a beneficial thing because it helps you to view your situation from another perspective. Sometimes, it can be healthy to laugh, even when things seem dire. It allows you to rest for a bit when things get really tough.

Bravery

Bravery is not the absence of fear but the strength to overcome what is causing it, even when every part of your being is telling you that you won't be able to make it. Bravery can come in many forms. In survival situations, it takes on the form of choosing to fight for your life when it would be much easier to give up. Bravery never backs down from a fight.

Motivation

Finally, we all need motivation. Motivation is the desire to carry on even when there seems to be no hope. It is a skill cultivated by pushing yourself to complete tasks even when you feel tired. It is the glue that holds your survival together. It can sustain you long after other tried and trusted methods have failed. Never give up hope.

Chapter 2:
Water: Where to Find It and How to Use It

It is a known fact that without water, humans will die after a very short period in the wilderness. Therefore, water is simply essential for basic human needs and cannot be ignored. The Rule of Three suggests the following theories.

Rule of Three divides significant aspects of survival into multiples of three. For example, humans cannot live for three minutes without air. You cannot live for three days without water, nor three weeks without food.

If you're in a group, you'll need to ration water according to how long your journey will be versus how many people are on the team. If it's just you, the situation becomes more straightforward. The key to water management is conservation. It would be best if you showed that you could plan ahead for several days and keep your supply going until the moment that you can be rescued. But first, you need to find and prepare the water, depending on where it is.

Where you can obtain water is mainly dependent on where you are in the world. Water is not readily available in the desert and thus must be carried along before entering the area. In the jungle, there are no such shortages. However, water may not be drinkable due to it being toxic, polluted, or filled with dirt or sand. If these issues are the case, then you'll need to bring a filter with you so that the water can be drinkable. In addition, you can make use of water purification tablets. Both of these things are necessary. But, in order to avoid putting the cart before the horse, let us look at the way in which you can procure water.

Finding Water

Water can come from many sources. The most common of these are rain, snow, lakes, rivers, and ponds. No matter where you are in the world, there should always be water available. Start by making sure you aren't wasting the water that you already have. Next, seek out other available sources of water. Remember, sometimes sources aren't apparent to the untrained eye. You will need to do your research before you find yourself in these situations so that you're able to find water when the time comes. The first thing you need to do is to be aware of the most common sources of water. These are areas that you can see and can easily access. Let us look at some of these areas.

Many people wonder if they should drink water at all if it is not clean or purified. The truth of the matter is that you will die a lot more quickly from dehydration than you would from water-borne diseases. Sometimes you have to make a choice on the spur of the moment. The best course of action, though, is to always look after your health. If you're prepared in advance, you stand less chance of finding yourself in these situations.

When you find a source of water, always assess it before drinking. Where is it situated? If it's a stream, does it flow downhill? If so, there may be contaminants further upstream that you're unaware of. For example, rotting animal carcasses and other waste can all contaminate water and make it unsafe to drink. Always purify and boil your water if you're able to. Never assume that water is safe to drink unless you can identify and know it is completely drinkable. With that being said, valleys are a great place to find water because water always flows downhill. You can use this to your advantage.

Lakes, Ponds, Streams, and Rivers

Always look for the most obvious forms of water first. When you find these sources, take a look at the color of the water. Dark, opaque colored, and still or slow-moving water is stagnant and might not be safe to drink. Water that has chemicals will have an unnatural hue and is definitely unsafe to drink. Water with chemicals in it cannot be made safe by purifying and boiling it.

Puddles

Water can be found in small depressions in the ground that collect rainwater and runoff water after storms and rain showers. You can also find this water pooled in crevices in rocks and caves, as well as in the hollows of trees. Don't drink water found in trees that are poisonous.

Always assess the water in puddles for signs of life and algae. If there is significant microscopic life living there, move on to other sources.

Rain

Rainwater is the best source of water you can find if you are lucky enough to have a shower. Unless rainwater has run off another surface on its way to the ground, it is perfectly safe to drink and is purer than other forms of water. Collecting rainwater can be done in many ways: through using plastic pots, using clothing items to collect water and many other methods of collection.

Digging a Hole

Digging a hole can sometimes yield water if you dig in the right spot. If sand is wet or if you can perceive water under the surface, you can dig down to reach it. Let the water slowly fill up the hole. If you're at the coast, dig on elevated ground in order to avoid accessing saltwater. Digging near patches of vegetation can sometimes yield a good amount of water if you dig to the right depth.

Dew

If there are known dew in the area, you can access this if you construct a dew trap. Dig a small hole in the ground and place a cup at the bottom. Cover the hole with clear plastic, secure the plastic in place, and you should be able to harvest some of the dew in this way. You can also lay a cloth on the ground to collect some of the water. Make sure to wring it out at dawn before the sun comes up, or the water will evaporate and be lost. Dew traps don't typically yield the most water. However, if the dew is reliable, it is an efficient way to get some water.

Distill Water

You can distill water in various ways, namely in a solar still or by boiling. If your water is undrinkable, place it in a pot over the fire. Boil the water using a cloth placed over the container the water is in. The steam will be caught in the cloth, and you can then wring it out and use it. A solar still can also be useful. Start by digging a hole in the ground somewhere where the sun's rays can strike it and reach the bottom of the hole. Place a few green leaves or some vegetation in the hole. Add a collection container at the bottom and cover the hole with a piece of clear plastic. Place a small rock or stone in the middle of the place directly over the top of the collection container. As the temperature of the hole heats up, moisture from the vegetation inside should start to condense on the plastic, dripping down towards the container.

Water from Plants

Plants are a great source of water as they store it in their leaves, roots, and fruits. However, knowing which plants to take water from can be tricky. Some contain water within their stems and shoots, such as bamboo. Others, such as different kinds of trees, contain water within their roots. Grate or grind up chips of wood from the roots of the trees until it is pulp. As the water seeps out, catch it using a container. Some tree roots might give more water than others.

The aforementioned bamboo is one of the best natural sources of water you can find and should be used at every available opportunity if it is present in the environment. When you find it, look for the thicker stems that sound like they have water inside them. These will usually be hollow. Make a notch about four inches above the joint in the stem and collect the water that runs out of it. You can use this water without having to worry about purifying it as it will be fresh.

Cacti are another fantastic source of water and are probably one of the best-known sources of water. There are many different kinds of cacti, all of which grow in harsh and dry environments. Not all cacti can be used for water, however. The great Saguaro cactus of Northern and Central America, for example, contains liquid that is toxic. All cacti contain milky fluid that must be avoided, except for specific varieties. Cut the cactus open so that the inner flesh is exposed and suck out the liquid. You can also make pulp with the interior of the cactus by mixing up the flesh inside, as this will produce more water. However, this should be avoided as it can kill the plant. Always try to respect the environment, even if you are in dire need of water.

You can collect water from plants in indirect ways, such as condensation. Simply place a bag over the top of a plant and tightly seal it by the stem. In a while, if there is sunlight, you'll see water droplets start to form on the surface of the bag. You can use this water immediately as it is perfectly fresh and safe to drink.

Sea Water

Seawater cannot be drunk immediately as it contains too much salt. It will poison you if you drink more than even a tiny amount, as it changes the pH of your blood and causes organs to stop functioning the way they should. Seawater must be distilled to remove the salt, but this is a laborious process for little reward. If you find yourself in a desert island survival situation, it may be tempting to take huge gulps of seawater when nothing else is available. However, this is a fatal mistake. Allow your common sense to take over, and instead, carefully gather water in other ways. These ways won't make you sick and won't lead to lethal complications.

Other Signs of Water

Vegetation is one of the biggest indicators that water is nearby. Clusters of trees, bushes, and plants are surefire signs that water is at least below the surface of the Earth there and that water has been in that region in the recent past. Look for signs on the earth that water flowed there. Valleys, where there are bunches of trees, are great places to find water. A lesser-known way of finding out where water is is to look at the sky. The patch of sky over a water source will often appear bluer than the rest of the sky. In addition, dawn is a great time to look for water. Fog and mist tend to congregate over water sources.

Wildlife Indicators

One of the most common ways to track water sources is to look for animal spoor or footprints. However, these are not the only ways that you can make use of animals to find water sources. First, look for signs of animal waste. They will invariably point to water sources since many animals leave their waste near sources of water. Birds are another excellent indicator that water is nearby. Low-flying, grain-eating birds could be an indicator of water. The presence of enormous swarms of insects inside cavities such as a tree trunk could be an indicator that water is inside. You can use a plastic tube to siphon the water out of these cavities. Finally, use your ears and listen for the presence of water-dwelling animals, such as frogs and toads. They can lead you to water sources if you can hear them in the distance, particularly at night. All you have to do is follow the sound.

Unusual Water Sources

If you find yourself in a winter situation and snow and ice are on the ground, you can make use of these. However, before you get tempted to scoop up handfuls of snow, bear in mind that it will have to be boiled and purified as well. Depending on the climatic and environmental conditions, snow might contain impurities. You can melt snow over a fire, but you can use your body heat to do so in the absence of this. You can also make use of tree ice if snow is not a viable option. However, be careful of ingesting the water from tree ice if the environment is susceptible to pollution or there has been a recent nuclear fallout.

How to Determine Water Quality

There are numerous ways you can tell if the water in a specific area is safe to drink without even testing it. Obviously, you want to boil and purify all water if you can. But if you're in a hurry and you cannot wait, there are some indicators that can, at the very least, give you a sign that water is reasonably safe to ingest. These signs apply not only to the water but also to the environment that the water is in. Look at the types of animals that are living in the water. What kinds of animals are they? Certain kinds of frogs and fish will only live in water that is fresher. You can research what these specific animals are, but, in a more general sense, water that is teeming with healthy aquatic life is generally more fit for humans. Water that is covered in algae, muddy, green, or stinking is not generally water you want to ingest, even if you boil it and filter it. There are some chemicals and substances that can't be removed from the water so easily. Always ensure that you're able to trace the source of where your water comes from so that you can assess whether there are any contaminants in it.

Finding the Cleanest Source Possible

Realize that clear water doesn't necessarily mean that it is safe to drink. In prepping situations, you need to ensure that the sources of water you bring onto your property are clean and safe for you to drink. Make sure that the place you decide to pitch your survival home is close to sources that are not contaminated. Always look for sources of life in and around water sources. A lack of life means sources may be tainted. A green and algae-ridden stream may be putrid, but it means that there is life in the water. If taken and used, and prepared correctly, this water can be drunk once it is in a safe state. Always filter, boil and treat any and all wild sources of water, no matter how clean you think they may be. Always verify that there are no bacteria in the water by looking at the state of the area where it has come from. And finally, never assume it is safe before you try it.

Purifying Water

Once you've obtained water, the next step is to make it drinkable and safe for consumption. If you're using it for other purposes, it is not such a big deal if the water contains contaminants because these aren't getting into your system, i.e., if you're washing or bathing in it. But if you're drinking it, you need to take the utmost care. So, what are the ways you can purify your water and make it safe?

Boiling

One of these ways is by boiling it. Boiling gets rid of the impurities, but it doesn't get rid of the larger particles. If you're able to get a fire started, boiling is a relatively simple process:

1. Filter the water through a clean cloth.

2. Draw off the clear water.

3. Let it boil for about 3 minutes and leave it to cool before drinking it.

Water Purification Tablets

Water purification tablets are a valuable thing to have when you need to purify water in a hurry. They do not, however, remove particles from water. This can only be done through filtering. The best tablets to use when purifying your water are iodine tablets. These are cheap and easy to find. They do, however, leave a certain taste in the water. Different brands of tablets last longer than others. Always check the shelf life of the tablets you're buying. A product called *Potable Aqua* is one of the best products you can buy because it purifies water in a very short space of time, in about 35 minutes. When you don't have time, and you need to purify water in a hurry, this can be a great product to buy. However, if you have thyroid issues or allergies to shellfish, you might want to avoid using iodine if at all possible. Children also dislike its strong medicinal flavor.

Filtering

Filtering is a great way to get rid of particles, dirt, and insects from your water. It will also remove sand and grit. It is easy to set up because you can use natural materials, such as rocks and stones. Filtering water through sand itself will remove many of the impurities, but you will still need to boil it afterward. Create a cone out of leaves or twigs or some other kind of material and fill it with sand, small stones, or vegetation. Place a piece of material or fiber at the bottom of the cone before you do this to prevent your filtration material from leaching out. Boil and wash your cloth before using it as a filter.

Distillation

Distillation has already been addressed in some detail, but you should know a few more helpful things about it. Distillation is a technique used in the tropics and the Pacific, where the climate is humid. Often, you'll discover water in these locations that seem safe to drink, but it is, in reality, fairly bad for you because it contains large amounts of salt. One way you can get rid of this salt is through the process of distillation. As mentioned previously, you need a container and a source of heat. Heat the water in the container with a cloth over the opening of the container. As the steam rises, it will be trapped in the fibers of the cloth, which you can later wring out and use. The residue from the water should be left behind.

Chemicals

You can use chemicals to purify your water, such as bleach, but this process should be approached with great care. Bleach is among the most common disinfectants used to purify water. A few drops are sufficient to purify a moderate amount of water. After adding the bleach to the water:

1. Put the cap back on your bottle and turn it upside down, unloosening the cap, so a little of the bleachy water gets out onto the rim of the bottle.

2. Allow some of the water to get onto the outside of the bottle as well.

3. Leave the bottle in a cool, dark place for about 30 minutes.

It should taste like chlorine and be perfectly safe to drink.

Plants

You can make use of various kinds of plants to purify your water. Banana peels and fruit peels are among some of the most accessible plant materials that you can use. Place the water in a bag or container and tightly seal it with the type of plant material that you want inside. Chemicals within the plant itself will naturally disinfect the water. Be extremely cautious if you're in the wilderness and you don't know what specific plants are present. Some could be deadly poisonous and should be avoided at all costs.

Build Your Own Filter

You can construct your own water filter using a few bits of wood and some flexible hose and glue. It is a straightforward project that will really help out if you're in a pinch. A piece of PVC pipe is attached to a water source, and glue or epoxy is used to secure the wood inside the tube. Water is then passed through the tube and filtered through the wood on its way to the container or receptacle you are using. This is a great way to filter your water, and it is safer than some other methods.

Now, when living in a prepper situation, you're going to have constant sources of water flowing through or near your property, or you should have if you have chosen the right location for your home. Depending on the way you have chosen to set up your water purification system, you're going to need to keep other methods on hand for emergencies. This is part of your long-term planning phase. One of the best ways to prep for water purification emergencies is to keep a steripen. They are small and easy to use, and they can prep up to 8,000 liters of water. This is a tremendous amount for something so small. They should be an integral part of any prepper's arsenal.

Chapter 3:
Don't Starve: Finding Food in the Wild

The Importance of Food

Food is the next most important element in your survival journey. Without it, you can't hope to stand the rigors of the environment, and it provides the much-needed energy and sustenance in a harsh and unforgiving landscape. In this section of the guide, you'll learn about where to find the food that you need, what the best kinds of food are for you, and how to prepare such foods. It's important to be aware of how to cook and store food once you're in the wilderness. The knowledge contained in this chapter will allow you to pick out the right equipment before embarking on your survival journey.

Food provides energy, which is vital once you're on the trail. Without it, you could quickly fade away and not have the strength to do essential tasks that will help you to stay alive. Food provides a morale boost, and it is a great distraction from the difficulty of the situation that you find yourself in. Food is absolutely vital to life in the wild. It is of the utmost importance that you receive the vitamins and nutrients that your body needs to stay healthy and strong while in the wild.

The essence of hunting is to try and find the food that is the most accessible first. If you spend more energy hunting for food than the energy you will obtain from it, then your efforts are being wasted. Therefore, efficiency is key in the wild. Part of this efficiency consists of planning ahead so that you can be prepared for any kind of eventuality.

In an off-grid home situation, you'll need to plan ahead because you won't have access to meat at a butcher unless your home happens to be near a market. Therefore, you will need to know how to hunt, kill, prepare, and store meat so that it doesn't go bad. In addition, by storing said meat, you're saving up for the future.

Where to Find Food

Food of many different kinds is all around you. You just need to know the best places to find it based on the environment that you find yourself in. Let's look at some of the places you could encounter on your survival journey and how these differ in terms of the food you can expect to find and also how you can access it.

Wetlands

Wetlands are home to a huge variety of life because they contain large bodies of water, as the name suggests. In these bodies of water, you can find all kinds of life. Animals from all over the region come to drink at these water sources as well, and this means it is much easier to track and trap prey. Examples of these water sources in wetlands include ponds, lakes, streams, and rivers. You can find frogs, toads, fish, mollusks, crustaceans, and snails in these areas. In addition, aquatic life can be located in the muddy bottoms of these rivers, streams, and ponds.

Near the ocean, eating is even better. Various kinds of fish, crabs, mussels, clams, and seabirds all present an excellent opportunity to grab something to eat. Tidal pools are a fantastic way to find prey that is trapped when the tide goes out. Always be sure to be careful what you eat and ensure that it is not poisonous.

Valleys and Mountains

Inland areas can contain both mountainous, rocky regions, open fields, and forests. One of the most accessible sources of food you can come across in these regions is insects, such as grasshoppers, locusts, and crickets. Termites, ants, grubs, and other similar creatures can be found in rotting plant matter, logs, and vegetation. Frogs, salamanders, birds, eggs, and worms can also be eaten, but caution is needed with some kinds of frogs and salamanders that can be toxic to humans. Eating these kinds of animals won't cause you to gain weight or provide a sufficient amount of energy, but they will keep you alive in the short term. It is about making use of what you have when you are able to find it. There is no room for sentiment when you're faced with a potentially perilous survival situation.

Deserts

Food is typically harder to come by in arid regions due to the lack of water. Desert areas are more of a challenge to find any kind of protein source because there are fewer animals that live there due to the extreme dryness of the climate. Finding food in these regions can be a challenge at the best of times, and so you have to take what you can get when you can find it. However, there are certain kinds of animals that have found a way to exist in these regions, despite all odds. These include yak, various burrowing squirrels, and rabbits, among others. Snakes can and have been eaten in the desert. They are a good source of protein when there is little else to be found. Scorpions are also present. They may not present to be the most glamorous source of food, but they will help you to survive when there is nothing else. Be careful of hunting them. When you encounter one, hold it down with a sharp stick and remove the tail. Next, peel off the shells, and roast them over a fire. Insects and various kinds of burrowing lizards are also common in these regions. These can be treated the same way as you would the scorpion: split small lizards open, remove their internal organs and roast them over a fire with a sharp stick. There are numerous ways to prepare insects, which will be addressed later in this guide.

There are a number of key problems you might face when hunting for food in the desert, and it is best to be prepared for this. The first is that animals that live in these arid regions are often well-camouflaged and adapted to protect themselves if they are faced with danger. As a result, they are difficult to catch because they are well suited to a lifetime of avoiding capture by larger predators. The second issue is that time able to be spent hunting for food is limited because of the inhospitable climate.

Tips for Finding Food in the Wild

These are some helpful tips for finding food in the wild and strategies for planning your approach to finding food before you even embark on your survival journey.

The first tip you need to be aware of is to avoid brightly colored creatures, as these are colored in such a fashion as a warning to predators. These animals can contain bitter substances, toxic chemicals, or spines or hairs. They can also bite or sting. This does not mean that all brightly colored animals are dangerous, but that the vast majority are.

Before you go out, do your research thoroughly so that you know where to find food and what to expect in any survival situation. Although you might have the right equipment, this doesn't mean that you will be able to use it effectively. Therefore, you need to plan ahead thoroughly and use your knowledge wisely.

Carrying various guidebooks can be an invaluable help in survival scenarios. However, you might not know everything about the subjects you most require an understanding of. In these cases, you will need to get a book that helps you to access and use this knowledge on the spot. Great examples of these guides include plant guides and guides to different kinds of animals familiar to the region you will be traveling to. Plants, in particular, need special attention, as there are many varieties that look like each other. Educate yourself on plant identification before going into the wild.

Always remember that unless impossible, you need to cook all food thoroughly in order to eliminate pests and diseases. Cooking food also makes it more palatable and pleasant to eat. In addition, the warmth acquired from hot food can raise morale, so before you begin your survival journey, always be sure you know how you are going to generate heat and power so that you can cook your food thoroughly.

If you're going into the wild, you're going to need to know how to hunt and kill various forms of wildlife. While it would be nice to find food laid on, in the wild, the initiative is required in order to gain the food you need for eating. Therefore, you have to be prepared to trap, hunt, and catch animals, birds, and fish. Educate yourself on proper methods of trapping and the tools you'll need to take along with you in order to construct said traps.

In emergencies, you'll need to have this knowledge stored. What will you do if there is a sudden food shortage and the shelves are bare? Money will profit nothing. Only your knowledge of the wild will matter because you'll be equipped to take advantage of the conditions around you. Having a general understanding of how to find food starts with being prepared and being educated. With that being said, let's look at the most important foods that you will need to be going for and what you should be looking to hunt and eat based on your skill level in survival situations. Not everyone has the skill to go after the same food. Some people are more experienced. You should not spend unnecessary energy seeking after large game, for example, if you do not need to be doing that. Rather focus on things you are able to manage.

Pyramid of Wilderness Survival Food

What is the Pyramid of Wilderness Food?

Knowing what food you can and can't hunt for and trap in the wild is vital to ensure that you don't waste time going after the wrong kinds of prey. Doing so will result in wasted time and precious energy that you can't afford to lose in a precarious survival situation. So, to avoid this problem cropping up, there is a chart to help you plan your hunting, fishing, and trapping escapades. It is known as the pyramid of wilderness survival food. The pyramid categorizes your ability to hunt and catch prey based on your survival ability. This could save you time and also your life because you won't be going into situations you can't handle. In addition, this pyramid will explain the techniques used to obtain certain kinds of food, examples of the animals you will be looking for, and how to cook and prepare these foods.

When you first begin your survival journey, you'll be looking at the most basic of foods you can find. You'll be eating food that consists of slow-moving prey and animals that are harmless and easy to catch or food that doesn't move at all. These kinds of food include plants and insects.

As you become more skilled, you'll graduate to fish and faster-moving creatures. At your most skilled level, you'll be chasing and trapping quicker and larger prey in more complex survival situations. Some foods may seem strange to you, given their position on the pyramid. One of these foods you wouldn't expect to find high up on the pyramid is mushrooms. This is because mushrooms take a lot of skill to identify, and so they should be left to those preppers and survivalists who are more adept at identifying those that are safe to eat and those that aren't.

At the highest level, you'll not only learn to kill large game but to skin and prepare it as well. This requires a knowledge of how to prepare different kinds of meats in different situations.

Tiers of Wilderness Food

Large Game

Large game is right at the top of the pyramid, as it represents the most difficult prey to kill. It requires specific kinds of weaponry and more sophisticated traps than other forms of creatures. These animals are best left to expert survivalists. Examples of these kinds of animals are larger herding animals, such as elk, gnu, yak, caribou, deer, wild boar, and other similar creatures. Note that the animals on this list are not only reserved for the experts because of their size; they are also extremely dangerous if they are threatened. Hunting these creatures requires the use of a large caliber weapon that could draw unwanted attention to yourself. Hunting with silent weapons is difficult and requires patience. However, hunting and killing are only the beginning steps of the process. You need to know how to prepare, store, and carry the meat once it is killed.

Every species of animal is different, but for the most part, when you are faced with large game, you need to approach it in much the same fashion. First, make a small hole at the top of the breast and allow internal gasses to emit. Be prepared for a foul odor. Next, remove the entrails. Make an incision along the carcass to the pelvis and open up the abdominal cavity. Cut away the internal organs and put them in a bag if you're intending on keeping them. Do this as quickly as possible because entrails left inside the carcass could make the meat toxic. Try as much as possible to keep the meat in a cool place so that it degrades less quickly.

Turn the carcass upside down and allow the blood to drain out. Be sure not to let any waste matter from the animal to come into contact with the meat, as this can cause it to go sour. Next, remove the intestinal tract from the back of the animal and use the "hole" at the back end as a draining vent for internal juices.

When you want to cook and prepare larger animals, you'll need to be aware of how to set your cooking station up. Again, this should have already been thought about and prepared for before you even started hunting and killing specific kinds of game.

For cuts of meat from large animals, you will want to build a spit that can be used over a fire and rotated. There are various ways to do this. A green stick works well over an open fire. Affix the cut of meat to the stick and place it over the fire using two forked upright sticks to hold it in place. Turn the meat at intervals to keep it from burning. Alternatively, you can use a similar arrangement to hang a fireproof pot or another container above the fire, and you can boil your meat in stock or liquid. What you decide to do with it depends on the time you have and the resources you have available to you.

Smaller Game and Birds

Next on the tier list are birds and smaller game. These creatures are high up in the tier list because they are difficult to catch, and they require a certain amount of effort to trap and hunt down. They are, however, not as difficult as hunting the largest game. A lesser experienced hunter might have success with these animals, but it will require a considerable degree of survival and hunting skill. Knowledge of how to construct snares and traps is necessary in order to be successful at this level of hunting. Examples of the creatures you'll be hunting in this tier are quail, ducks, pigeons, geese, rabbits and hares, mice, squirrels, and similar creatures. Try to stay away from hunting creatures like weasels and badgers, as these animals are highly aggressive and could do more damage to you than you know before they die. Avoid potentially painful situations.

Prepare small game and birds by splitting them open down their belly and opening them out. Remove the entrails from these animals. Remove the feathers from birds and roast them whole without removing the bones. Save the heart and liver from these birds, as it makes good eating. When preparing pheasant, partridge, pigeon, grouse, quail, and other similar birds, leave them in a bucket of water for a few hours in order to drain the blood from them.

For small animals, like rabbits and muskrats, for example, you can hang them up by their legs in order to drain the blood. Make two small slits at the ankles and make two slits in the inner thighs that connect to the vent and throat of the animal. Pull off the skin and try to leave it as intact as possible. Open up the animal and remove the entrails, saving the heart and liver for later. In muskrat species, remove the scent glands from inside the animal, as this can taint the meat.

You can cook the birds or small game over a spit, or you can simply lay them on the hot coals. What you can do is to let the fire burn down until only hot coals are visible. Then take several green sticks and lay them on top of the coals. Place the birds or game on top of the coals and allow them to cook gently. You can even make kebabs using pieces of the meat. You can attach various kinds of vegetables and other meats to these kebabs.

Storing meat can be done through a process of salting and drying it. The first key thing to note is that meat needs to be stored in a cool and dark environment. Too much sunlight and warmth will proliferate the growth of bacteria in uncooked meat. Cooked meat can be stored for a short period of time without preservation, but it must be consumed as soon as possible after the animal is killed.

For longer-term storage, the meat will need to be sun-dried. First, trim off the fat and cut the meat into long strips. Hang these strips in the sun until they are black and hard. Meat can be kept in a bath of saltwater before this process in order to cure it. When eating dried meat, be sure to eat another kind of food alongside such, preferably something that contains fat in it. This will avoid you getting an upset stomach.

Other sources of nutrition you can gain from both small and large game are their bones, organs, and blood. This may not sound like the food you're used to in your urban environment because this is a different and altogether serious situation. When you're faced with life or death situations, you have to use every part of the animal, including the parts you might not be used to seeing.

Animal blood is a rich source of iron and many other nutrients. When an animal is draining, be sure to have a container ready to catch any blood you might want to use. To make it more palatable, add it to a broth or soup.

Bones are rich in minerals. You can grind them up, or you can add them to soups and stews as an accompaniment. Crack open large bones using a heavy object and extract the marrow from them. You can use this in many different ways, and it is highly nutritious.

Reptiles, Amphibians, and... Mushrooms?

The next on the tier list are reptiles, mushrooms, and amphibians. These creatures are slightly easier for survivalists to find and trap, but they still require a reasonable degree of hunting skill and definite knowledge of more than just the basics. Finally, mushrooms are high up on this list because specific knowledge is required in order to identify which are poisonous and which are edible. An inexperienced survivalist would not be able to identify these mushrooms with any degree of consistency.

Reptiles and amphibians can be split open and their insides removed. They can then be lightly charred over an open fire. Be careful of any poisonous varieties.

Amphibians can be caught using your bare hands. Frogs, toads, turtles, tortoises, and other similar creatures make great eating and are easy to catch. They can be cooked and roasted over a fire. Turtles can be boiled in their shells. Detach the shell before eating. Cut the heads of scorpions and snakes along with their stingers. Be extremely cautious when gathering certain varieties of frogs as these can be deadly poisonous.

Edible varieties of mushrooms can be eaten raw or cooked. They can be added to other dishes and make a great accompaniment to soups and stews. Each variety is unique in its texture and flavor. However, always be sure that the variety of mushrooms you choose is safe to consume. Do your research thoroughly before attempting to gather mushrooms from the wild.

Seafood and Eggs

The following creatures on the list are crustaceans, seafood, fish, and eggs. Eggs are easier to find since they don't run away when you try to catch them, but they still require a certain level of skill to safely remove them from their nests. Fish requires reasonable skill to catch, but it can be easily and quickly learned. More inexperienced survivalists will be able to handle these creatures when searching for food efficiently. All that is required is the knowledge of how to make fish and crustacean traps, the knowledge of where to look, and the knowledge of what kinds of fish and shellfish are safe and edible.

You can catch fish and other seafood by making a hook. Cut a piece of stick about 2 inches long and sharpen it at both ends. Hide the small fragment inside a piece of bait. When a fish swallows it, it will become lodged in its throats.

The way to prepare fish is by simply roasting them on the grill or splitting them down the middle, removing the backbone and entrails, and laying them over hot coals. Depending on the size of the fish, you might not need to even debone or clean them. This is the case, particularly with fish-like sprats. They don't need to be cleaned, only quickly roasted over hot coals and eaten as quickly as possible. You can, of course, gut these small fish if you wish, but they are often eaten as they are. For larger fish, you do need to gut them, but it is a relatively simple process. First, cut the fish from the tail side to the head on the belly side. Pick the fish up by the tail and remove the scales by scraping them off. Remove the bloodline and the kidneys from them.

For storage, you can dry the fillets of fish over a fire on low heat. Again, make use of some kind of material to make sure they don't get burned.

Mollusks require certain knowledge in being able to prepare them. Always bring a short, sharp knife with you if you're going to be trying to gather mussels, scallops, winkles, and similar creatures. These creatures survive by clinging tightly to rocks in shallow pools, and they need to be removed. Simply cut through the muscle holding the creature to its surface, and it should dislodge. In order to open bivalves, as this is what these are known as, cut through the hinge at the back of the creature, applying pressure to the point. Then, pry it open and extract the creature inside.

Insects

Insects themselves can be prepared by removing their spiny legs, wings, heads, and hard shells and only eating the body itself. For those who are squeamish about the idea of eating insects, a good way to make them more palatable is to grind them between two stones. Then, you can use their remains in other dishes, and you won't notice that you're eating them. Avoid eating poisonous or toxic insects, such as ticks and flies, as these can make you sick. These are valuable kinds of foods to come across, but you need some knowledge of which are edible. So, this tier is for those who are novices but who have taken a few steps down the road, as it were. It is not the most accessible tier because it still contains a level of skill when you're trapping and collecting insects.

Insects can be prepared in many different ways. Remove their heads, wings, outer carapaces, and legs, and impale them on sharp sticks before roasting them over the fire. Worms can be prepared by removing their guts and lightly roasting them. They can be soaked beforehand to get rid of any internal matter. Worms can also be eaten raw if desired. However, be careful with doing this as some can harbor parasites themselves. Do prior research on what can and can't be eaten.

Nuts, Seeds, and Grains

The second-largest tier of the pyramid contains the foods considered to be among the easiest to find, harvest, and collect. Unsurprisingly, this tier contains much of the food belonging to trees and plants. Fruit is on the list, as well as nuts and grains.

Nuts, seeds, and grains can be eaten raw or cooked. They do not need specific preparation other than removing the outer shells from certain varieties. Some kinds of nuts, such as acorns, need specific kinds of preparation before they can be eaten and should be avoided. But, for the most part, nuts and fruits make an easy and nutritious meal.

Plants and Berries

The last tier is the widest and therefore considered the easiest. These foods include berries, roots, tubers, flowers, and shoots. Finding these foods is an entry-level skill for survivalists and should not be too taxing. Some education is required, but by and large, if you're in this tier, you should stick to only eating the foods that you are able to collect and safely prepare. Fruit and other kinds of plants can be eaten raw for the most part.

Chapter 4:
Staying Warm

Why Staying Warm is Important

Staying warm in colder weather is vital to survival when you're in the wilderness. There is no doubt at all about that. Cold weather, torrential rain, sleet, snow, and fog can all combine to ruin your morale. Therefore, it is vital that you have a plan of action for when this kind of weather comes along. You need to be prepared both mentally and physically to handle the rigors of climate. The way you stay prepared is by researching and understanding how to stay warm and dry even before you find yourself in such situations. When electricity and heating fail in urban environments, how will you keep yourself warm? You need to be already prepared for such an eventuality. Cold weather is not the only killer. Rain and floods can also prove potentially fatal. How will you deal with such events and ensure that you stay warm and dry?

The Dangers of Cold

Cold is not only damaging to morale, but it is also a killer blow to your health and wellness. Cold causes various functions in the body to stop working properly. It can further weaken a body already wracked by the pressures of life in the wilderness. Humans were meant to thrive and survive at optimum temperatures.

In order to effectively plan for all kinds of weather conditions, including cold, you'll need to be aware of what you can and can't bring along with you on a trip. You have only a certain amount of room, and therefore what is carried must have a specific purpose. The dangers of not preparing for freezing temperatures are manifold.

Your body will start to feel tired and sluggish at first. Your alertness will diminish, and your mind will feel less clear. Because you feel sluggish, you won't have the energy to get up and perform critical tasks that you need to survive, such as finding food or water.

Brain fog is another key danger of extremely cold temperatures. When the body cools down, your metabolism slows, and blood cools as well. As a result, less oxygen is imparted to the brain, and your thinking slows down as a result.

Shivering and shaking are one of the signs that the temperature within the body is too low and needs to be raised urgently. In addition, shivering can mean that you won't be able to carry out specific tasks that require you to be articulate, such as tying knots and other crucial skills.

Frostbite is the bane of those who find themselves mired in extremely cold conditions. When water molecules trapped within the body begin to freeze, it causes damage to internal organs, skills, and nerves, among others. It can even cause death in rare cases when decay and gangrene start to set in. The early stage of frostbite is called frostnip, and it is a warning that more severe problems are about to occur. Therefore, you should take measures to keep the affected part of the body as warm as possible when you begin to experience these symptoms. Usually, frostbite is most dangerous when it affects the body in conjunction with other symptoms.

The following are the signs of frostbite: numbness in the affected area, discoloration on the skin, a feeling of pins and needles, itchy or sweaty skin, or a clammy feeling, a loss of sensation to cold or heat, a hardening or lack of plasticity in the skin, pain, and soreness in the affected area, and other symptoms.

It is important to note that at first, your skin won't feel hardened at all, so this is not a reliable indicator of incoming frostbite.

When you notice these symptoms, the first thing you need to do is to try and keep the affected part warm as much as possible. Gently warming the area will help to alleviate the pain and inflammation.

Hypothermia is another nasty condition, which is well known to experienced survivalists. This infamous condition occurs when the body temperature drops below a certain level, and your bodily organs can't work properly as a result. Death can occur in a matter of hours if not treated. The body has an optimum running temperature, and falling below this temperature can be fatal in many circumstances.

Symptoms of hypothermia include the following: shivering, slurred speech, faint pulse, irregular breathing, trouble articulating sentences, poor coordination, memory loss and confusion, and eventual loss of consciousness. It is incredibly challenging to deal with hypothermia if you're alone because of the way in which it affects the body. Therefore, you need to be around people who can help you. Or even better, prepare for your survival experience and take the necessary steps to keep yourself warm. Let's start by looking at the most basic of needs when you're in the wilderness: the shelter itself.

The Need for Shelter

This section is not so much concerned about learning how to build a shelter in detail, as this will be addressed a bit later. Instead, it is concerned with the need to start preparing yourself by gathering the tools and materials you'll need before you start your journey and what knowledge you'll require in order to build an effective shelter. In short, it is about the strategies you'll require once you start planning for the long term.

Strategies for Dressing Properly and Shelter Building

Dressing For The Cold

Having looked at some of the dangers associated with cold weather, let's look at some of the ways in which we can get out of the cold.

The first strategy is to stay dry by any means necessary. The rule of thumb when you're in the wild is that moisture on your clothing or next to your person at any time is a definite no-no. Moisture destroys your equipment, food, tools, weapons, and clothing. In addition, it can make you uncomfortable and lead to rashes and skin conditions, which can be really distracting and frustrating when you're already in a difficult situation.

Dressing yourself correctly so that you make the best use of warm air pockets is a good way to stay warm in cold and wet conditions. This is done by layering clothing so that it wicks moisture away from your skin. Outer layers can be used for protection against the wind. Wear clothing with spaces in between the linings so that warm air circulating through the fabric from your body is trapped between the layers. In doing so, you'll keep yourself warmer than if you were just using simple fabrics, such as wool, for example.

Invest ahead of time in clothing that can keep you warm and dry. Think about what fabrics you'll need in order to create such clothing, in case you're unable to get any. For example, fur-lined jackets are a must if you live in an area where potentially cold weather is a common occurrence.

The buddy system is the means by which people who are in survival situations together keep each other warm and dry. It is always good to have someone with you when you're in these situations. They can help you with situations you can't cope with on your own, and vice versa. For example, sleeping back to back with two blankets over the both of you can help you to maintain more body heat.

Use leaves as insulation. This is a strange idea to the inexperienced person. But, it makes perfect sense to the survivalist because leaves form a protective layer around the person and can be tightly packed together. These leaves can be packed inside clothing or close to the body as a means of insulation.

During the day, you can find a thermal face, such as a sun-warmed rock, tree, or even the ground itself, and position yourself so that your body is perpendicular to it. By doing so, you'll gather the rays of the sun.

Getting dressed is still your best way to insulate yourself against the cold. Place the tightest layers against your skin to transfer the moisture produced by sweat away from your skin. Sweat is meant to cool you down, and you definitely don't want that happening when you're in the wilderness. Sweat can quickly turn to ice and leave you with hypothermia. As the temperature increases and decreases, remove or add clothing when it is required.

Make use of foil blankets, as these absorb heat and keep you warm while you're huddled underneath them. In some cases, these foil blankets can be used inside clothing as an added layer of protection. Buy a number of these blankets ahead of time and store them in your home in case you require them for you and your family.

It's important to know what clothing to pack before you go on your journey. The right kind of clothing can make or break you once you're in the wilderness. If you know you're going to spend time in colder climates, you'll definitely want to adjust your wardrobe accordingly. So, what clothes will you want in your luggage? Choose clothing that is lightweight, as you will be carrying it. Avoid heavier fabrics unless they are necessary. The following fabrics work well in cold climates: wool, synthetics, and puffer jackets (and similar items of clothing). Woolen socks and gloves are necessary if you want to keep your extremities warm.

Shelter Building

Whatever kind of weather you find yourself in, you're going to be required to build a shelter at some point, even if the weather is not cold. If it is, you need to construct a shelter that suits your needs and keeps you warm, dry, and protected from the elements. Part of the long-term strategy for survival involves educating yourself about building different kinds of shelters in various types of environments. Let us now focus on the shelters you're going to need to build in colder climates.

Natural shelters are a great way to get out of the elements if you're lucky enough to find them. When you're in the wilderness, you have to make use of whatever you can get when the need arises. So, a natural structure that can protect you is a very fortunate thing to discover. These shelters usually take the form of caves, hollow trees, and other types of overhanging vegetation. But what do you do when there are no such shelters, and you're left to face the elements alone? You need to put your survival strategies into practice.

A tarp survival shelter combined with a fire can keep you warm in cold climates. But how do you make such a structure? Start with an A-Frame structure. Tie a string between two trees that are close to each other. Drape the tarp over the string, making sure to weigh the edges down with heavy rocks and stones.

If you don't have any tools or resources and a tarp is the only thing available to you, you can wedge yourself inside the tarp, and it can keep you warm and dry. Simply wrap the tarp around yourself, making sure you are as well-covered as possible. The heat from your body won't escape, and it will circulate around the interior of the tarp and keep you dry and warm. Stuff the interior of the tarp with leaves, moss, and other soft and dry vegetation. Lying directly on the hard ground will cause you to lose massive amounts of body heat, and thus it is imperative that you insulate yourself properly when you sleep.

Building A Fire

Building a fire is one of the most important skills you can master and should be practiced before you even embark on your survival journey. Being stranded in the wilderness without having a fire is a death sentence, particularly in cold climates. Building a fire not only keeps you warm, but it discourages predators, raises your morale, allows you to heat water and cook food, and many other necessary benefits.

There are various ways to construct fires so that it offers you the best kind of warmth. Knowing what specific ways you can build a fire will be advantageous to you in the long run. Depending on your circumstances, you will need to adjust your fire-making strategies. Your tools are also incredibly important in determining what kind of fire you're able to make. If you have a flint, for example, you're far more likely to be able to get a fire started quickly than if you have only matches and the surrounding area is wet and damp. If it's raining and cold, you'll also need to think about how you are going to approach the process of fire-making. Fires need warm and dry environments. If you don't have access to these types of areas, or they are not readily available, then you will need to move to an area where you can build a fire under cover. There are a few key things you need to be aware of before starting a fire.

Choosing a Location

When choosing where you build your fire, you need to consider its position in relation to other flammable materials. If you're carrying anything that could conceivably catch fire, you need to store it properly so that it doesn't leak. But this aside, the most important thing to be aware of when selecting your fire location is that it needs to be in a well-ventilated area. Make sure that nothing is in the way of the fire that you intend not to burn, such as food supplies and cooking materials. Keep your fire close to the source of the materials you intend to cook. For example, if you want to boil water, it would be a good idea to build your fire near a river so that you don't need to worry about walking many miles to fetch water. If your fire is for a signal, then build it in an area where it can possibly be seen by a passerby. If you want to keep yourself warm, build a fire in an area where heat won't escape but where oxygen can still permeate. The moral of the story is to build your fire in the area that best suits your needs at the time.

Gathering Tinder and Kindling

There's a difference between tinder and kindling, which many inexperienced fire starters may not understand. But it is important to understand the difference between these two things in order to start a fire effectively. Tinder refers to the small, dry objects, such as twigs, leaves, and grass that are used to set alight the larger objects, the kindling. In other words, tinder is the catalyst that makes kindling burn. Further examples of tinder are moss, pine needles, pine cones, and many others. Finally, kindling are the logs that make up the fire itself or whatever you are going to use to keep the fire going.

Constructing a Fire Pit

Constructing a fire pit will allow you to keep your fire confined to a specific area. This is a good idea if you're intending on spending a lot of time in a specific area. The first thing you need to do is to remove all debris and dirt from the area that you're going to use. Next, arrange your stones in a circle, like a cairn. In the center of this circle, arrange your sticks in a teepee-like structure. This is going to be your kindling. The next step is to arrange your tinder. Place the tinder in a bunch at the bottom of the kindling so that it surrounds it. Light the tinder, and you'll start your fire.

Ignition

When speaking of lighting your fire, there are various ways to do this. You can start your fire by using a flint to create a spark, but there are many other ways to do this as well. Which method you use depends on what tools you have at your disposal. Let us say that you are equipped with only basic survival equipment, with no fancy items in your inventory. Let's look at some of the methods that are commonly employed to start a fire.

The first is called the bow method, when you make use of a simple friction system to simulate the action of a drill to create heat, and therefore a spark. You will need several items: a simple bow, a string, a handhold, a drill, a board, and a knife.

For the board, you'll need to find a branch that is about 6 inches across. Make sure that the wood is dry and not green or wet, or you'll never manage to make a spark. Trim the branch until it is about 1 foot in length. Split the branch in half and make sure that you trim it down so that it is about 3 inches across. Cut a small depression about 1 inch from the edge of the board and about 5 inches from the end of the board. Cut a small wedge out of the board in line with the depression you just made.

For the handhold, whittle down a 5-inch-long, 3-inch-wide piece of branch and trim the edges so that it can be used safely. Next, cut a notch in the center of the wood piece.

For the drill, select a stick of a similar length to the handhold. Next, whittle down a piece of the branch until it is around 0.8 to 1 inch thick. Sharpen the dowel at both ends, but make it sharper at one end than the other.

Choose a string or a shoelace, whatever you have available, which should be about one-quarter of an inch in diameter.

Find a thin, bendable, but strong piece of wood to use as a bow. It should be around three-quarters of an inch in diameter.

In order to assemble the drill:

1. Apply pressure to the board with your foot on the opposite side of the board from where you cut the depression earlier.

2. Wrap the string around the drill, making sure it is held securely.

3. Make sure that the string is between the bow and the drill.

4. Hold the handhold in your left hand and press your left wrist to your left chin.

5. Cap the depression in the handhold over the top of the drill and stroke the drill back and forth while pushing back on the handhold.

6. Continue until you start to see small sparks and then start to gently blow on the area to generate oxygen in the flame.

When it starts to burn slightly, add the lit tinder and continue to provide oxygen to the area.

Extinguishing a Fire

When you need to extinguish the fire for any reason, you need to starve it of oxygen. This can be done in various ways. Bear in mind that the only time you want your fire to go out is if you are finished using it. In the majority of cases, if you will be trying to get warm, you definitely don't want your fire to go out unless it dies naturally. However, if you need to move in a hurry, you're going to want to extinguish your fire quickly. If your fire for some reason starts to get out of control or sets something else on fire, you need to think quickly. Trample on the burning kindling and embers if they have died down a bit. Or you can also scatter the embers, grinding them into the dirt to deprive them of oxygen. In the event that the fire is large and cannot be trampled, move the pieces of kindling away from the base of the fire so that they cannot feed the fire anymore. It should soon die down.

Chapter 5:
First Aid

In the current state of our world, getting a small cut or a minor abrasion is no big deal, given the resources that we have to treat such incidents. But, what if you found yourself in a situation where you did not have access to such resources? A small cut in the wild can turn into something much more serious if it is not treated. Minor issues become major ones when the ability to treat them efficiently and safely is removed. At times like these, you will really need to think seriously about your strategy for first aid. What are the tools and equipment you'll need for first aid? What can you carry on your trip? What are the most vital items you'll need in your pack? You also need to make sure you understand the skills required in order to care for someone else or yourself on the trail. These skills must be learned and honed before you head out onto the trail. In this chapter, we'll look at what your preparation must include by looking at the basic techniques you need to know.

The situations where you're going to be required to use your skills are in survival situations, natural disasters, and times when the risk of loss of life is high, and there is a significant risk of injury or death. There are specific skills you need in order to be able to be of service in these situations. Let us look at some of the skills that you will need to learn as part of your preparation.

Necessary First Aid Skills

There are three specific skills that are required in order to effectively administer first aid. These three skills all focus on certain areas that are critical to emergency situations. These skills are stopping a wound from bleeding, stopping someone from choking, and more. Generally, the skill of being able to think on the spot and being resourceful. This is not a skill that one can usually just master. Instead, it is training your brain to think in a certain way by practicing coming up with solutions to problems you face on a daily basis.

One may think that CPR would be the most critical skill that one needs to learn when first starting to learn first aid. However, CPR will only keep you alive for a certain amount of time until proper help can arrive. It is vital to treat the source of the problem and to attend to it with urgency.

What are the most important tools you need for first aid in a survival situation? What is the one piece of equipment you can't do without? This might be different for other people, but there are specific items that are invaluable and those you need to invest in while you are preparing for your survival escapade.

The most important item you need to carry is actually within you, your mind. Your knowledge and preparation for a situation can serve you better than any item you could carry.

Apart from this knowledge, there are items you can carry with you that will really help you out in any emergency. Let's look at some of these items. Create a bag with these items before you leave.

Gloves are important because they protect you from potentially harmful substances, and they can prevent the spread of infection or contamination of wounds. Latex gloves can fit most sizes.

SAM splints are useful because they are flexible and can be used in many different circumstances. Elastic bandages are great to have around as they can fit over many different kinds of cuts, sprains, and abrasions. They help to reduce swelling and improve the stability of injured areas. Always be careful of circulation issues when dealing with bandages. The goal is to try and make the area safe and secure, not cut off the blood supply.

Scissors, cloth, tape, and other similar items are also needed. You can customize your bag as and how you need it, depending on the circumstances you will find yourself in. Duct tape is invaluable in survival situations. It can secure any bandage in place, temporarily stop blood flow, repair footwear, and be placed over areas that require protection in order to stop blistering from occurring.

Common Household Items for First Aid

Packing a first aid kit for a survival trip need not be an expensive trip. Many items lying around your house can be used within your survival kit. The key to finding these items is to be creative and to make the best of what you have in your home.

Cloths

Cloth can be cut from various kinds of fabrics. Depending on what you intend to use them for, these cloths can be absorbent, clean, or porous, allowing air to penetrate through to a wound. For example, T-shirts make great clothes and bandages in a pinch. Avoid materials such as denim, as these tend to not be as absorbent.

Liquids

Liquids, such as water can be used to clean wounds in an emergency. Make sure the water itself is clean so that there is no risk of infection to the affected area. Any other kind of clean liquid will do, as long as it does not present an adverse effect on the injured area.

Duct Tape

As previously mentioned, duct tape can be used to close wounds and to bind up injured areas. Be careful with latex tape, though, as some people can be allergic to it. Not all wounds need to be bound. Some need to be exposed to oxygen in order to dry and heal properly. Deeper cuts may require stitching, depending on the severity of the injury. In the rare situation where a body part is severed for some reason, expert medical attention may be required. Always assess the situation and see what you are capable of and what you can achieve within the context of the given situation. The most important first aid resource you have available to you is knowledge.

Skills Everyone Should Learn

Broken Bones

Broken bones are common in survival situations. They can occur when there are trips and falls, as well as in various kinds of accidents. The main concern with a broken bone is that it might shift into a potentially dangerous position. The key issue, therefore, needs to be the securing of the bone in place. If a fractured bone shifts accidentally, it could press against a blood vessel or a nerve and damage it. This could impede blood flow and potentially damage a limb long-term. If the fracture is open, it could lead to infection. The first step is, therefore is to deal with this open wound. Once the wound is closed, the bone needs to be secured.

CPR

There are seven steps that must be followed in order to do CPR correctly. The first of these steps is to position yourself correctly over the body. Make sure that the patient's body is on a flat and secure surface. Next, place the heel of your hand over their chest and make sure that your fingers are interlocking. This means that you keep your arm straight, cover the first hand with your other hand and make sure that your fingers are crossed. Next, you need to give chest compressions. Lean your body forward so that your shoulders are directly above the patient's chest, and press down on the chest for about two inches. Release the pressure, but don't take your hands away, and allow them to come up. Repeat about 30 times every minute; that is to say, once every 2 seconds.

Open the patient's airway by tilting their head back slightly and opening their mouth. Next, lift the chin up to open the airway.

Pinch the patient's nostrils closed with two fingers and support the patient's chin with the other hand. Take a breath and place your mouth over the patient's mouth. Next, blow into the patient's airway until you can see their chest begin to rise. Remove your mouth from the patient's mouth and watch to see if their chest is rising. Repeat the last two steps again once. Repeat the series of chest compressions thirty times, followed by two rescue breaths. Repeat these steps as long as is necessary or until help arrives.

Heimlich Maneuver

The Heimlich maneuver is used to help those who are choking. Choking occurs when a foreign body enters the throat and blocks the airway, hindering breathing. In such situations, urgent attention is required. First, stand behind the person who is choking. Next, wrap your arms around their waist. Next, curl your hand into a fist and place it underneath the navel of the person. Pull your fist back sharply directly in an upward motion, and the object should be dislodged.

Cleaning and Dressing Wounds

Cleaning and dressing wounds is a situational task

because it depends on the nature of the situation and the wound concerned. If a wound is superficial and not bleeding much, you don't need to be as urgent with your treatment. On the other hand, if a wound is bleeding excessively, it may be an indication that there is an underlying artery or vein that has been severed, and urgent help is required. If the wound is superficial, treat it in the following way:

First, wear gloves to avoid the risk of infection. Next, make sure the wound is clean. Scrub it gently with a gauze or cotton pad, along with soap and water. If there is anything stuck in the wound, remove it with a pair of tweezers without causing too much discomfort to the victim of the injury. You can also pressure-clean a wound without touching it by using a syringe. Next, make sure that the water you use is disinfected. This can be done with iodine tablets. Finally, apply pressure to the injured area using a clean cotton or gauze pad in order to get the bleeding to stop. If it turns out that the injury is more serious than you first thought, more extreme measures may be required.

After cleaning the larger wound, you need to bandage it. This may be necessary in the case of smaller wounds as well, but they generally only need a lighter dressing. Apply antiseptic ointment to the bandage. Next, wrap the wound gently but firmly. If it is a non-adhesive bandage, you may need to use duct tape to secure it or use a safety pin. If the dressing becomes wet or dirty, you need to change it. Be sure to check it every day. If a joint is injured, you may need to splint it. After the wound is bound up, check the patient's ability to move the injured part without pain. If they have some mobility, it is a good sign that there is blood flow to the area. If they feel numb, the bandages may be too tight. Loosen them a little, or remove them and reset them.

Treating Shock

Shock is a condition that can occur when there is severe blood loss followed by a drop in blood pressure. If you're unable to stop the bleeding from a severe injury, then you might need to administer shock treatment. Lie the victim down gently on a comfortable but flat surface and raise the affected or injured limb above the heart so that the blood begins to flow back towards the heart, putting less pressure on it. Make sure that the victim is breathing. If not, administer CPR immediately. Loosen any tight-fitting belts or clothing. Make sure that the victim is warm. If the victim is choking, endeavor to remove the obstacle from the airway to clear it. If the airway is not clear, turn the victim on their side.

Stopping Bleeding

In order to stop bleeding, it is essential that you raise the affected part so that it is higher than the heart. It is vital that you prevent that wound from bleeding and cause excessive blood loss. Another way to avoid or stop blood loss is to apply pressure to the affected area. Still, another way is to apply a tourniquet to the affected limb. By doing so, you're restricting blood flow and giving the wound a chance to clot.

Treating Hypothermia and Hyperthermia

Hypothermia is a condition whereby the body loses heat to such an extent that it is unable to function. Hyperthermia is the exact opposite. Both conditions can be potentially fatal. But how do we treat conditions where the internal temperatures of the human body are not working as they should? There are various precautions that can be taken in order to safeguard ourselves against these conditions. But if they fail, we should be prepared to adopt measures that can raise or lower our body temperatures as necessary.

In the case of hypothermia, handle the affected person gently. Move them out of cold zones and into a more protected area. Cover them with blankets or whatever you have on hand so that their body heat doesn't escape. Monitor the person's breathing and feed them hot drinks if necessary. If they do not improve, seek more expert medical attention.

In the case of hyperthermia, a person needs to be made cool and should be moved out of heated zones, such as direct sunlight. Move the person into a dark and cool environment, and fan them with towels. Administer a cooling drink and administer ice packs to various parts of the body in order to reduce their internal temperature.

Treating Burns

Treating burns can be complicated by the nature of the

injury and what caused it. The first thing you should do when you encounter someone with a burn of any kind is to remove the source of what caused the burn in the first place. Next, assess the nature of the burn. A 1st-degree burn is a burn that only impacts the exterior layer of the skin's surface. A 2nd-degree burn penetrates the deeper structures of the skin and causes noticeable damage. Third-degree burns cause long-lasting damage and are the most serious burns of all. They require urgent medical attention.

For first-degree burns, place a cold compress over the burn and secure it in place. You can use various substances such as burn cream to try and treat the burn. Soak the wound and take a painkiller if needed.

For second-degree burns, more urgent action is needed. The top of the skin's surface will be blistered and damaged. Keeping the area clean is paramount. A light dressing can be applied. The worse a burn is, the longer it will take to treat.

For the most serious of burns, the third-degree burn, intensive medical treatment may be required given the extent of the burn and its position on the body. There is the myth that these kinds of burns are the most painful due to their severity. However, this may not be the case as many of the nerve endings in the skin and below the skin will have been seriously damaged. So there may be no feeling in the affected area. When encountering such a burn, seek expert medical attention, make sure that clothing does not stick to the burn, and do not attempt self-care. Raise the injured part above the heart if possible. There is no timeline for healing for a burn as severe as a third-degree burn, but without help, serious scarring can occur.

Concussion

A concussion occurs when the head or skull is subjected to trauma, leading to brain injury. A concussion is a very serious condition, as it may look like everything is normal to the onlooker, but severe bleeding or damage may have occurred inside the brain. Rest is one of the best treatments for concussion, despite advice to the contrary. What should be observed are signs of confusion, dizziness, or lack of ability to complete simple tasks. If there are signs of more grave brain damage, expert medical attention may have to be sought. For the most part, the patient needs to be kept calm and well-rested. If there are external head injuries, treat them in the normal way as best as possible in the given situation.

Making a Splint

Making a splint is done so that broken bones can rest and recover without being jolted out of position. It also lends strength to the affected limb and keeps it straight so that bones don't recover in a crooked position. Splints can also be used for limbs that are sprained or dislocated. At its simplest, a splint is just a piece of wood, metal, or plastic, or another stiff material that is tied to the affected limb to prevent further damage to it. Depending on the materials you have, you can make your own splint.

First, control any bleeding if there is a need to do so. Next, place an amount of padding over the wound and secure it in place. Finally, place the splint under the injured area and secure it in place. Be sure not to put too much pressure on the injured area or press on it.

Dehydration

The first signs of dehydration are dizziness, lack of concentration, and profuse sweating. When you see these symptoms, you need to immediately assess whether you've been drinking enough water during the day. If you're doing physical activity, you're going to lose more water, and therefore, you need to drink more. Dehydration isn't always noticeable at first. But this is the danger of being dehydrated. You're not always aware of when you are getting to this phase. Therefore, it is imperative that you take the proper precautions to avoid finding yourself in a bad situation. If you're far from home and find yourself in a desert or a compromising situation, you'll need to try and think of a way to get water when more obvious solutions aren't available. One of the options available to you is called a hydration bladder. This is a kind of plastic bag with a sleeve inside of it that helps you to store water and insert it into the victim's mouth if they are unable to physically swallow. Fluid is accessed through a hose attached to the bag. The cure for dehydration of any kind is to drink, but if you are unable to find water and have passed out, or you are unconscious, more urgent medical attention may be required.

Chapter 6:
Defending Yourself in the Wilderness

Why is Learning Self-Defence Necessary?

The idea of self-defense may not have crossed your mind before. It is tempting to think that you will always be alone and never encounter any kind of opposition or criminal element. However, you need to be prepared for anything and everything. All circumstances must be prepared for in the planning phase of your trip.

Situations You May Encounter

The situations you may encounter depending on where you are going. Often, you might not encounter any kind of situation where you need to fight while you're in a survival situation. But, in everyday life, you may encounter these situations. Therefore, you need to be both mentally prepared and physically ready to combat the threats that you encounter and to minimize risk to both yourself and the people you love. In order to be fully prepared, you need to learn the techniques that will enable you to get away safely. But what are the situations you might encounter where you need to have these techniques ready? It can be daunting to think that you might be called upon to engage physically with someone in order to protect those you love. But knowing when and where these situations might occur can make the situation a little easier.

Criminal Encounters

Encounters with criminals can take place anywhere and at any time. But there are some situations that are riskier than others and where you need to be more aware than ever. We live in a society that is unpredictable, and danger can strike at any moment. People are desperate, but they don't show it immediately. What will you do when people are hostile towards you and demand your possessions or threaten your loved ones? Start by taking evasive action.

These criminal encounters usually take place in areas that are not well-lit. Walking alone at night with possessions is an open invitation to being accosted. Avoid areas that are of poor repute. Be particularly careful in places where you would normally expect to be safe. Such areas include public parks, restrooms, and other similar sites. Criminals know where people will let their guard down, so you need to think differently than you usually would if you want to stay safe. If, however, you take all the necessary precautions and still end up in a situation where you need to defend yourself and others, you should only use these defensive techniques as a last resort. The skills described in this chapter are not to be used for aggressive purposes but to give yourself enough time to escape from the situation. They are meant to provide enough time for you to make a quick getaway without being harmed and losing your possessions.

Encounters with Wild Animals

In some cases, you might be required to defend yourself from wild animals, particularly in a survival situation. Self-defense techniques may or may not be effective against these animals, but you can still prepare by learning techniques for avoiding them and techniques for engaging with them, and what weapons work best against certain kinds of animals. Some techniques you can use when facing aggressive wild animals are standing tall and appearing intimidating. Don't back off, even if this is your first instinct. And certainly don't turn tail and run away, or turn your back to the creature. Many predators would consider this a sign that the chase is on. Instead, always stand still, adopt slow, deliberate movements, and never take your eyes off the creature. When we face these creatures, we need to, for a minute, step outside of our own human body and think the way an animal does. What would intimidate them most of all? What would cause them to be more aggressive? Think about how other creatures would view you and tailor your behavior accordingly. It might just buy you enough time to save your life.

Self-Defense Techniques

There are a number of techniques you can use when you find yourself in a situation where you need to defend yourself. These techniques are mainly for when you find yourself unarmed, but they can be used in many other types of situations. Knowing how to protect yourself is about more than just knowing what moves to use in any given situation. First, you need to know the correct areas to aim for. Second, you need to be physically strong enough to strike out at those areas in a way that will injure your opponent and give you enough time to make a clean break.

Above all, remember that the best form of defensive technique is to prevent the incident from happening before it occurs. By being safe, you're avoiding having to face the incidents in the first place.

Basic Techniques

These basic techniques cover the wrist hold, the front and back choke, the bear hug, the mount position, and how to land a basic strike. It is essential that you practice these techniques over and over again so that when it comes time to use them, you will be primed and ready to do so.

There are some preliminary moves that you might want to learn so that you can use them before you find yourself in a tight situation. For example, when someone approaches you that looks hostile, you need to draw attention to the situation as much as possible. Criminals hate people who make a lot of noise and disturbance, as it draws attention to their activities. Try to get as much in the face of the criminal as possible. They hate it when people stand their ground against them. If you have a loud whistle, blow that too. These tactics are not guaranteed to keep you safe, but they do serve as a way of attracting attention to the situation the attacker was trying to keep as secret as possible.

There are a few weak points you also need to be aware of. The main points of an attack should be the eyes, nose, throat, and groin area. Always target these areas first as they are the most sensitive, and they feel the most pain.

The eyes are a great point to attack first because they are sensitive and, if an attacker can't see properly, he can't reach you. You have the upper hand immediately. Striking at the eyes is the most important point you can reach.

A strong and determined strike can easily break the nose, and if not broken, at least seriously injured, leading to all kinds of complications for the attacker.

A blow to the ears of an attacker can render them stunned for a few moments, allowing you to get away. This is because the ears are responsible for helping us balance due to the number of tiny hairs they contain. A strong strike to the ears causes disorientation.

A blow to the throat can cause severe pain and discomfort for an attacker for a few moments. If the blow is a strong one, it can even disable them for a while as they struggle to catch their breath. Therefore, when you strike, it should be with your palm. Your fingers should be held straight and tightly against one another, and the blow should be short and sharp.

Other important areas you can attack are the center of the torso, the knees, and the groin area itself. The groin area is particularly painful because there are many nerve endings in this area. As a result, it can wind an opponent for quite a long time, giving you enough time to get away safely.

Biting is an effective way to get an assailant to release their grip, particularly if a part of their body, such as their arm, is near your face, and they happen to be holding onto you at the time. Many people might be put off at the idea of biting someone, thinking it is in some way unhygienic or dirty. But the reality of the situation is that you have to do whatever is necessary to save your own life and protect those you love in any situation you encounter. Sensitivities have to be put aside when you are fighting for your life. So, when you bite, bite hard and with all your force. This should surprise the attacker enough for them to let go momentarily, so you can make an escape.

Grabbing the little finger of an assailant and twisting can be enough to make them let go in some cases. It is a surprisingly painful maneuver that can catch an attacker unaware. Make sure you grab onto the little finger, bend it back and twist it. The attacker will have no choice but to let go, as you can break his finger if he does not.

The wrist hold is a technique used by an attacker where they try to control your arm by grabbing your wrist. You need to regain control of your arm so that they can't strike out at you. Countering this tactic will change the momentum of an attack, and it can be employed in order to use an opponent's momentum against them. What if the attacker grabs you by the wrist.? What do you do next? What you need to do is to find the weakest point of the wrist. This is usually the region between the thumb and forefinger. Try to rotate your arm so that the momentum of your arm is pushing against the weak point of the attacker's hand and lever yourself free. Don't try to pull or kick back against the opponent because this will lead to you losing your stable base, and you will be easier to knock off balance. Always keep a firm footing.

The front and the back choke is a technique used when the attacker grabs you around the neck and back but leaves your arms free or grabs you from the front and has their hands around your neck. It may not seem like an advantageous position to be in, but if you keep a cool head, you can turn the tables on your opponent. Place one of your forearms on the attacker's and use the other hand to push back against their throat. Make sure to push hard against their throat with your fingers and use your full force.

The bear hug is an attack from behind where the attacker grabs you and pins both of your arms to your sides. Without the use of your arms, what do you do now? Well, you use your legs. Raise your foot so that it is almost parallel to the attacker's shin and stamp hard with all your force, raking the attacker's shin and damaging their foot in the first place. The initial shock, pain, and surprise might cause the attacker to loosen their grip for a fraction of a second so that you can make a clean getaway.

The mounted position is the most effective technique an attacker can use against you, and it is the most difficult hold to break out of. In this position, an attacker usually has you on the ground with their knees on your chest, making it extremely difficult to move or adjust your position to one where you can gain the advantage. But, there are still moves that you can make in order to reverse this seemingly impossible situation and still come out on top. The first step is to remain calm and assess your options. Next, turn on your side, bringing your elbow and knee together underneath the attacker's leg that is closest to you. Continue pushing against their leg with yours. When you read the half guard stance, that is to say, your opponent's leg is tangled with yours, turn on your opposite side and place both hands against the opponent's other leg. This should cause the opponent to be thrown off the stable base. Free both legs from underneath the attacker's control and use them to lever yourself away. There are many techniques that you can use to escape this most difficult of situations. The most important thing is to remain calm and stay prepared at all times. Use your innate ability to improvise and strike hard when the situation demands it.

Basic strikes are the bread and butter of any self-defense kit. If you're not as strong physically as you think you should be, you can still make use of these techniques to help you out in a difficult situation. They can be brandished by anyone, even those who have a slightly smaller frame. The key to their success is the technique, not outright strength. The following are some of the strikes you can use in different situations and how you can use them.

A heel palm strike is a common technique in self-defense situations. Standing in front of the attacker, strike towards the throat with your palm up, your wrist flexed, and your fingers strong. Recoil your strike once it meets its target, as this will cause the attacker's head to snap back. Striking the ears can also stun or disorient an attacker.

Fighting Dirty

When you're in a survival situation, there is no time to think about whether you're being nice to the other person, and there is certainly no time for sympathy. So in order to get the advantage and get away quickly, you need to adopt the same tactics as the criminals. In other words, in order to outwit a criminal, you have to think like a criminal. This does not mean that you turn your morals off. Rather, it means you are able to predict what they will do, so you can counter it. Sometimes this counter tactic may involve something like a groin attack. In this case, you need to be prepared to act in ways you wouldn't usually, given the seriousness of the situation.

One of these techniques is biting. It has already been addressed here, but you should perhaps know a few other things about this tactic. First, you need to make sure that any force you use is proportional to the attack that was used on you so that you don't get into trouble. Remember, your only objective is to escape, and this should be the goal always.

Eye gouging is another attack that can temporarily take

the momentum away from your attacker. Scratching or clawing at the attacker's eyes can be effective because it stops them from seeing your attacks and being able to attack you as a result. In addition, they might not know where you are because they're temporarily blinded, and you can escape as a result.

As the name suggests, groin attacks are attacks where you strike the groin area of an assailant. This is often the most sensitive area of the assailant, and it can cause them great discomfort. Make sure that when you strike these areas, you hit with all your force and don't hold back your strike at all. Strike and strike hard. You need to give yourself enough time to escape.

Using Weapons

Sometimes, the threat you face is more significant than you can manage to overcome with your own raw physical strength, technique, or power. At times like these, you need to rely on an equalizer to try and balance the odds more in your favor. To be clear, the use of weapons is never encouraged for the purposes of terrorism or violence and should only be used for defensive purposes and as a last resort. Weapons are a way to tilt the odds more in your favor and should be viewed as such. You want to immobilize or stun the attacker so that you can get away. You do not want to use more force than is necessary. There are many weapons, both designed for use and improvised, that can really help you to get out of a difficult situation. Let us look at some of these weapons.

Bags, shoes, keys, umbrellas, torches, and many kinds of household items can all be employed against the face of an assailant to teach them a lesson. Always be bold and never back down if you have to use these weapons. The only way to win is to be confident.

There are more conventional weapons you can use to protect yourself as well, such as guns, knives, and mace sprays. However, each of these things has its own advantages as well as disadvantages.

Mace sprays are effective at close range, but they can be used against you if you're not careful. They are also highly dependent on being accurate. However, if you do manage to deploy them, they can be highly effective at doing their job. They blind an opponent for a good length of time, which can be extremely useful in a dangerous situation. However, against multiple opponents, you are better off using other strategies.

Knives are cheap and simple to use, but they are the tool of an aggressor most of the time. Therefore, be extremely careful how you employ them. Usually, they are a killing weapon, and that is something you do not need to be doing. Before you decide to use one, you need to ask yourself whether you'd be prepared to physically stab someone. It can be a difficult ethical choice, and perhaps, these are best avoided as far as self-defense situations are concerned unless you absolutely have no choice.

Guns are even more ethically challenging. When you own a gun, it is usually because you intend to use it. And unless you are used to using such weapons, they can present a myriad of ethical issues. For example, would you be prepared to shoot and possibly fatally wound another human being? Do you have the knowledge and the skill to use them in potentially stressful situations? If the answer to any of these questions is "no," then you should probably not be investing in a gun for self-defense purposes.

How to Cope in Difficult Situations

In potentially difficult situations, knowing what to do can be challenging for even the most ardent prepper or survivor. Stressful situations always seem to challenge you in ways you never thought you'd be challenged, and there is always the gray area in which these situations seem to occur. Let's look at some of the situations you might be expected to encounter that require you to be mentally and physically prepared. However, life is about developing strategies that will aid you even before you face these situations.

When faced with multiple attackers, what strategy will you employ? You need to know that going down to the ground in such a situation could be a potentially fatal move. Always stay on your feet, and utilize this knowledge in any and every situation that you face.

When attackers are invading your home, and there are intruders inside it, or when you come home from work one day, and you realize that there is someone inside, what will your reaction be? You could call the police, but what would be the better solution? Maybe there is no time to call the police, and you have to make a split-second decision. Making use of household items can really save your life in this situation. Baseball bats, kitchen knives, brooms, axes, anything can be used as a weapon if you have the ingenuity to use it. If the attack is at night, resist the temptation to turn the lights on and instead operate in darkness. You know your own home better than anyone else, and turning on the light will only give the enemy unnecessary clarity. You're most effective when you're hidden and unknown.

When faced with an assailant with a weapon, you need to know how to act. First, try to stay out of range of the weapon and, if possible, grab it and try to control it. Once you've alleviated the threat to yourself, you can calm down and take control of the situation in a more effective manner. You can distract the assailant by dropping something, such as a purse or wallet. When their gaze is diverted, you can grab it and make your escape. But your reflexes have to be very quick in order to do this. The main thing is if there is another option to take that doesn't involve fighting back to save yourself, then take it, even if it means giving the crook your valuables. Your life is worth more than temporary possessions.

When you're faced with a riot, you need to keep calm and not allow yourself to be carried up in the state of emotion that is sweeping the situation. If you are not part of the riot, the easiest solution would be to get out of the vicinity as quickly as possible. But what if you are surrounded? You need to try and stay safe, and the best way to do this is to actually blend into the crowd and not try to stand out. The more you stand out, the more you will draw attention to yourself, which is what you want to avoid if at all possible. Stay out of sight, draw as little attention to yourself as possible, and try to move with the crowd so that you don't get caught in the crush. When you spy an opening at the edge of the crowd, move on and get out of the throng. The best advice is to not attend events where it is likely there will be a riot. This way, you avoid the possibility of being caught up in a situation you never intended to be in. If possible, get indoors and off the streets immediately. Stay away from windows and open areas. Always stay safe and avoid dangerous situations before getting into them. This is called being proactive rather than reactive.

If you have the money, get self-defense training. It will really help you to become more confident, and it can save your life in a difficult situation. There are different kinds of training available, from beginner to expert. But by and large, the best kinds of training are those which focus on the basics and honing down your critical skills necessary for self-defense. Fancy kicks are useless and impractical when faced with real-life situations and are impressive only for show.

Chapter 7:
Building A Shelter

Why is Shelter Important?

Shelter is one of the most basic necessities next to water and food. Without it, you could perish in a matter of hours if the climate you're in isn't favorable. Shelter keeps you warm and dry, and it can protect you against a number of outside dangers, such as wild animals. This chapter shows you how to make solid and stable structures that can keep you warm and safe in any kind of weather. This chapter also shows you how to make shelters out of natural structures so that you don't even have to expend the extra energy. Overall, it is important to be aware of how to create these shelters because they are the most important part of your camp. Without them, you have no protection from the elements.

The Danger of Weather

Cold weather, as well as hot weather, can have a huge impact on what kind of shelter you're going to build. But before we look at the types of shelters you can build, depending on the weather, we need to examine what dangers the weather itself can pose to you.

Cold weather is a killer because it can lead to a variety of conditions that affect the proper functioning of the body.

Hot weather can cause dehydration and other harmful side effects. Wind and storms can make building shelter and finding food more difficult.

A Wide Array of Shelters

There are a wide array of shelters you need to learn how to build depending on the circumstances you find yourself in. Cold weather shelters are going to vary considerably from what you might build if you were, say, for example, in the tropics. Things like storms and natural disasters also have to be taken into consideration when building your shelter. There are suitable structures, and then there are some which are not so suitable. You need to already have these designs in your mind so that you can plan them when you find yourself in a wilderness environment. Let us look at some of these structures.

First, there are cold weather structures. These are structures designed to keep out the cold weather or wind and to keep warm air circulating inside. These structures are made out of natural materials, such as ice and snow, or they are made out of materials that are strong so that cold can't penetrate their fibers.

Warm weather structures tend to be made out of materials that are less sturdy but more able to allow cooler air to circulate around inside.

The shape of a shelter determines how effective it is at housing the occupant and how sturdy it is against the elements. You ideally want a shelter with a strong roof, but this might not always be possible in some conditions.

Therefore, you need to make the best and sturdiest structure with the materials that you possess. Sometimes, your shelter might be made more for convenience purposes. In such cases, you need to build a shelter that is going to be easy to pack up and move when the need arises. Simple shelters might just be a tarp over an A-frame structure. This can shelter you quite well on most nights. In more extreme conditions, though, or for longer-term expeditions, you're going to need to build a structure that will last you a bit longer, and for this, you will need the right equipment and tools.

How to Build A Shelter

So, what are the first things you should be aware of when building a shelter? Of course, there are a number of considerations, such as the positioning of your structure and the location of it. But the most important consideration of all is what kind of structure you're actually going to build. This is determined largely by the kind of situation you find yourself in. What is the climate like? What tools do you have on hand? What is the environment like? What is the terrain like? These are all things that have to be considered before making your shelter.

Location

Your location is dependent on where in the world you find yourself. In the tropics, you'll have to contend with hot and humid conditions, sand, and probably jungle-like terrain. In colder regions, it might be more mountainous, and you'll have to think about building a shelter that can keep you properly insulated. If you know where you are going beforehand, you can prepare accordingly. But if you are not prepared, and you find yourself thrust into a wilderness you know little about, you will need to rely on your prepared knowledge in order to know where the best position for a shelter is.

If the weather isn't too cold, consider building your shelter on higher ground. This will give you a great view of the surrounding area and enable you to assess the terrain. If the weather is colder, you'll want to be out of the wind, and so you'll need to build your shelter in a covered location, such as a place that is shielded by trees. Do not build in a ravine gorge if this is possible, as cold air tends to settle there at night, although this is technically situated outside of the range of the wind.

Shelter Type

A round lodge is a common structure in tropical conditions and in all kinds of weather because it is effective at blocking both extreme sun and cold. It is structured with a triangular angled roof with a hole in the top of it for releasing the smoke. The roof can consist of thatch or grass. This kind of structure has been used all over the world and is particularly effective in wetter climates because the angled shape helps to aid in rain runoff.

A ramada is a type of open structure that is suitable only for hotter climates. Its flatter roof provides ample shade.

The structure itself is simple, consisting of four flat posts with a fabric covering. If you are in the wilderness, you can make one of these shelters yourself if you need protection from the sun.

A double tarp structure is popular in the desert. This is a structure that consists of four even posts and a tarp folded double, fastened over the top of them. It can really help to deflect the sun's rays and keep you cool in the process.

Pick a spot that is well-shielded from rain and sun, as well as wind. This is easily spotted, but the ground that you choose also has to be level enough to build on. Avoid building on uneven or boggy ground, as your shelter may not stand. Make sure that the location where you build your shelter is easy to access and that you can reach important sources of food and water. Don't cut yourself off from the areas that you need to get to. Make sure that the area you choose to build on is not on an actual water source or wet or boggy. The wet ground can also harbor pests. Make sure that you do not build near sources where wild animals go to drink, or they could cause problems for you. Never build, say, for example, near a watering hole.

Knowing what type of shelter you will build is helpful because it can assist you in determining the best location. A-frame shelters need a specific kind of ground so that you can set up the structure. An A-frame shelter or a tent also needs a couple of trees close by each other. A parachute tent structure only needs a single tree.

Simple Shelters and How to Build Them

This is a short overview of simple shelters you can build without overexerting yourself and wasting unnecessary energy and resources. One of the more popular structures is called the "lean-to" structure. It is an angled structure that is simple to construct and can be built in a short amount of time. First, lay some objects such as large logs against another structure, such as a tree or rocky outcrop. Then, create an overhang for yourself using several of these logs. This is a crude but effective way to make a temporary shelter.

A cocoon is basically a pile of leaves, sticks, and grass that you sleep in the middle of. It may not be the most sophisticated idea ever, but it will serve you well in a pinch on a cold night where there isn't much time to make a shelter. Simply pile as much soft vegetation up in a pile as possible and dive into the middle of it. Cover yourself with what remains so that you're inside the middle of the nest. Make sure you can breathe or have a space for some air. The heat from your body will circulate around the nest and keep you warm all night. If it works well for animals and birds, then why not for humans?

Similar to the lean-to, a fallen tree can make a solid temporary shelter. Lean branches against the windward side of a tree that can bear their weight. You should choose the windward side so that the wind is not blowing against the structure but rather with it. Huddle underneath the logs after making sure that they are secure. If you can make a fire, you'll be warm enough to survive most cold nights.

Stretch a line between two trees low enough to the ground to lie under, but not too low. Place a tarp over the line so that both sides drape over it. Place rocks on either side of the tarp to weigh it down. In a few minutes, you have a tarp shelter with minimal effort. In the event of snow, place the line or cord higher up between the two trees, making a steeper, angled runoff. This will prevent snow from collecting on the tarp.

Making a Bed

You need a bed in your shelter (or your shelter can even be a bed in itself). Either way, you will need a space to lie down for the night because proper rest and sleep are vital to your continued survival in the wilderness. Sleep helps your body recover and repair cells. It is also vital to mental clarity and focus. Make a pile of leaves on the ground slightly bigger than your body and about 8 inches deep. Burrow into the middle of this and pile as much on top of yourself as possible so that you stay warm.

Natural Shelters

Natural shelters are invaluable in survival situations because they save you hours of work and expended energy. And, they can be stronger and more stable than anything you could ever build yourself. Examples of these structures are natural caves in the rocks. If you find a cave, you have stumbled upon the perfect kind of shelter. But there are a few things to consider. First, know if there can be any other inhabitants inside. Caves are often used by large mammals. Second, caves can be drafty. They can also be nasty and unpleasant places. But the protection they offer is invaluable. Be careful of parasites or diseases in these caves. Always be guided by your nose when investigating them. Sea caves are another form of shelter, but these can be extremely dangerous if the tide comes in. Pools of water can be a warning sign that all is not well. If you see these signs, get out and make for another shelter.

Fallen logs and trees also make great survival shelters if they happen to be positioned in the right way. They may not be as cozy as a hut or a tent, but they can still offer some shelter and a dry spot during inclement weather. The same could be true of brush or trees. These trees can offer protection from the rain or relief from the sun.

Hollow trees can also be used for shelter, and they provide a snug, warm spot that is surrounded by hard, impenetrable wood. Who could ask for a better form of shelter? However, one does need to be careful with these trees. Depending on their size, they can contain any number of venomous creatures and also bats. Hollow trees are rarely unoccupied, so be prepared to deal with whatever you find in there.

Rock formations and rocky overhangs can also be used as shelter. These are not the same as caves, as they can be simple rocky outcrops that are attached to the sides of mountains and cliffs. They can also be boulders that are stacked together to form a kind of shelter underneath.

They can be effective at sheltering you from the rain and sun, at least temporarily. Be careful, however, that these structures are stable. A rock slide or an avalanche can mean instant death if you're underneath these rocky overhangs. Once again, be careful you're not sharing your space with other wild creatures.

Tools And Materials You'll Need

You'll need access to logs, rope or string, nails, saws or axes, and some kind of fabric covering, depending on the type of shelter you're going to make. You may need a tarp or some kind of thatch material made of grass to make a roof. If you're in arctic or colder climates, you'll need to get hold of a snow saw, which you can use to cut blocks of ice. Having a hammer, screwdriver, knife, shovel, and other associated implements can also be useful, no matter what climate you find yourself in.

Let us look at some of the more specific tools that will assist you in creating a solid and secure structure. These can be purchased at survival stores and packed before you leave for a trip. Then, if you find yourself lost in the wilderness, you can use the equivalent of whatever you're able to find or have in your pack at the time.

A tact bivvy is a kind of sleeping bag crossed with a tarp. It is a versatile piece of equipment that you need to have in your pack when you go traveling, especially to colder climates. The difference between tact bivvies and sleeping bags is that the former can fit in the palm of your hand and is much easier to carry than a heavy and cumbersome sleeping bag.

A survival tarp is a kind of tarp that is specifically designed for survival situations and is thick enough to be used as a shelter or covering for a shelter roof. It is waterproof, durable, lightweight, and can be stored easily.

Paracord is a rope that is used for binding and tying things together. It is a durable form of rope that is resistant to most conditions and very effective at securing shelter parts together.

Building a Fire in Your Shelter

If you're in colder weather, it is essential that you keep warm and safe during this time. The first thing you need to do is to create a fire so that you can keep heat circulating around the structure. Make sure that there is a hole where the smoke can escape, but don't make the structure so open that all your heat can escape. However, you're going to run into situations where you, inevitably, can't build a fire. This is especially true if you're living in a shelter made of predominantly dried materials such as leaves, twigs, and bark. It is basically one giant structure made of tinder, which a fire will destroy very quickly. It is, therefore, necessary to be able to construct other heating sources without the need for a fire.

The first thing you need to do is to find two large rocks. Find a rock approximately the size of a bowling ball. This is going to be your heat source. Next, dig a small pit in the floor of the shelter, which is slightly larger than this rock. Next, find a flattish rock to cover the entrance to the hole you have dug. It should be big enough to cover the hole entirely. Don't take rocks from streams or other water sources, as these are likely to explode or crack if heated. Heat your pit stone in a fire for several hours and carry it back to the hole with a shovel. Do not touch it at this point, or you will receive a serious burn. Place it in the hole and cover the hole with the flat stone you collected. This setup should give you ample radiant heat to last for several hours and with a fraction of the risk, you get from lighting a fire.

Bad Places for Shelter

There are a number of places you should absolutely never build your shelter because doing so would lead to a risk of death or imminent danger or cut you off from important resources.

Don't build anywhere the ground is damp, as previously mentioned. This can compromise the integrity of the structure. Don't build at the bottom of ravines and gorges where you're trapped, have no freedom of movement, and are subject to cold air at night. Don't build on the edge of ledges and cliffs, as appealing as the view may be. Not only are you in danger there, but you're also exposed to winds and the climate. Another good reason for not building in a ravine is the possibility that your camp might be washed away if there is a sudden flash flood. If you need to get out in a hurry, you might not be able to do so. So, always consider every aspect of the environment you're in before deciding where you pitch your camp.

Different Kinds of Shelters for Different Kinds of Environments

It goes without saying that your shelter isn't going to look the same in the desert as it does in the cold wilderness. There are different specifications required for different types of environments. It's helpful to know what kinds of shelters work best in these environments so that you don't end up building a shelter that is completely inadequate for the weather that you find yourself in — unsuitable at best and potentially a fatal hazard at worst. Let's start by looking at cold weather structures. We've already covered some of these, but there are many variations on these structures.

In snow and ice, you want a structure that is going to insulate you from the cold. An igloo or quinzhee is the best way to go about this. A quinzhee is a pile of snow that is hollowed out in the middle, making a warm and comfortable shelter. Pile snow about 7 or 8 feet high off the ground. As you're doing this, include some straight sticks vertically in the roof area as a kind of support structure for the shelter. When the snow is piled up, round it off on the outside so it is smooth. As the snow hardens, it will form a thick, impenetrable layer. You can then burrow out the interior of the quinzhee and find your way inside. This should be done before the snow has a chance to go hard. You can make the quinzhee as big as you like, but be careful. Powdery snow is not suitable for making a quinzhee. It is likely to collapse, and if it does so, you'll be buried. Always use glassy or icy snow. Always make sure your structure is absolutely sound and secure before you go into it. Be sure that the outside of the structure is rounded so that snow runs off rather than settles on the roof.

You can also pile a bunch of clothing on the ground in a relatively round shape. Next, you can pile the snow on top of it so that it forms a layer above the clothes. Finally, you can burrow in and remove the clothes from inside, creating a kind of cavity you can use as a shelter. Make sure that the snow is thickly piled so that it creates a solid wall structure.

An igloo is similar to a quinzhee in shape, but it is composed of blocks of ice rather than snow itself. These blocks can be cut using a snow saw or a large knife. Use a stick to outline the shape of your igloo as you build. In this way, you'll create a structure that is balanced and stable. First, test the density of the blocks you cut in order to make sure that they are secure enough to hold the weight of each other. Then, carry on building concentrically until you reach the top of the structure, where you can leave a small hole for letting out the smoke.

Forests and mountainous areas lend themselves to the building of tarp structures. This is because there are many trees to facilitate this kind of structure. Forests and mountains also lend themselves to building lean-to structures. You can make use of the materials that they provide to use in your shelters. Leaves, grass, and branches from these regions can also be used to buff out the structure even further and to create beds and other forms of material. Let's look at some of the shelters that can be built in these regions.

First up is the debris survival shelter. This is a shelter that is built for the express purpose of being flexible. It is like a sleeping bag and a shelter all in one. Its disadvantage is that it cannot be lived in like a normal shelter, but it will protect you from all the elements:

1. Look for a flat patch of ground away from any deadfalls and make sure that the drainage around the structure is good and that the ground isn't wet.

2. Choose an area with good exposure to the sun so that your shelter collects the heat inside and stays warm throughout the day.

3. Find a solid log that is going to act as the main support beam of your structure.

Make sure that the support beam is solid and not rotten in the middle because if it breaks, it could cause untold damage to you.

Find and secure a forked tree and lay the log across it so that it forms an angled beam. Next, make sure that the angle of the beam is enough so that you can lie underneath it. You don't want to make it too narrow or too tall, or the warm air will not be able to circulate properly or escape entirely. Next, cover the beam with a piece of the tarp so that both sides hang evenly. Finally, spread and weigh the sides of the tarp down with rocks so that you have a crawl space to get underneath in the event of bad weather if you just need to stay protected from the sun and the elements.

If you don't have a tarp, you can make the roof using ribbed sticks, short logs, or reeds or leaves. Start by placing the logs for the frame next to each other, leaning against the main pole. Ensure that they are even and line up with each other. Secure each log to the mainframe and ensure that the other end is deeply rooted in the ground. When the frame is in place, place the roofing material over the framework and make sure that it sits securely. What kind of roofing material you put on your roof depends on what you have available and what the climate is like. In warmer climates, you're likely to use leaves because they insulate while allowing cool air to circulate inside the structure. They also keep bugs out. You can use this same type of structure in a jungle environment to repel insects and other small animals and to prevent them from entering your shelter. A mosquito net can be hung over the open areas while you're in the shelter so that bugs can't reach you while you are inside. This is particularly important in the case of situations where there are a lot of mosquitos.

A spider shelter is just a kind of structure that has a modified dome so that you can sit up in it. It is slightly more complex than some of the other shelters listed in this guide. The framework for this shelter looks like a spiderweb. The first thing to do is to find one long branch, slightly taller than you. Next, find several shorter branches which are going to form the basis for the framework for the structure. About four branches should do. Make a pyramid-type structure with the four branches and fasten them together at the top, like a tepee. Put one end of the longest branch in a position so that it pokes through the top of the structure. Secure all of these branches tightly. The longest branch will make the structure stable.

In the gaps between the poles, you will need to add in the material to make your structure secure. This consists of what is known as "debris," the sticks, leaves, grass, and vegetation that covers the structure and protects you from the elements.

Overall, forest and mountain structures are largely dependent on making use of wood to create frameworks and then building up the outside of the structure as you go. If you have the correct tools, you may not even need a tarp. Keep an eye out for natural forms as well, and never expend more energy than you need to. Every step in the wild when you're planning a survival shelter is vital.

In the final part of this chapter on shelters, we'll look at some types you can build when you're faced with hot and arid conditions. Here, you definitely don't want to keep heat in your structure. You don't want structures that absorb heat. Instead, you need structures that will reflect it. You will need structures that allow you to get shade from the sun's terrible rays and shelters that allow cool air in and circulation to occur. One of the more recognized kinds of shelters is known as the dugout shelter. This kind of structure can be implemented with great success in the desert because you're able to dig a hole in the soft sand, and you can form your shelter around this. In types of harder or rocky ground, this might not be possible.

You will need a shovel or a sharp object for breaking the hard ground or for digging. Both are preferable. You will need an axe for cutting branches if there are trees around. If not, you'll have to build the framework out of another kind of material. You'll need some kind of material for making the roof, such as leaves or grass. First, you need to find a spot where the soil is soft but still firm enough to dig a hole. This is going to be the foundation of your shelter. Dig a hole about 8-10 feet deep, depending on how big you want your structure to be. Leave a slope leading to the hole as a form of exit and entrance. Remove any unnecessary soil from the building site and deposit it somewhere else so that you don't attract unwanted attention. Try to make your den as inconspicuous as possible. Add vegetation to the bottom of the hole to make a comfortable bed. In the desert, you're not going to rely so much on being warm, but you do need to get out of the sun. In order to create shade, you can lay sticks flat over the top of the entrance and leave a small entrance for you to get inside. Once the sticks are in place, in an overlapping pattern, lay leaves or grass over the top of the sticks. Finally, cover the top of the structure with sand so that it looks as natural as possible. Although the dugout-style structure takes a little longer to build than some other structures, it can really help you to remove cool and in the shade while in arid environments. The most important thing to remember in any desert situation is to keep cool and out of the sun's harsh rays, so pick any shelter that helps you to do that.

Having a Backup Shelter

At some point, if a natural, economic, or financial disaster hits the world or even your area, you're going to have to think about how mobile your current system of living is. If there is danger in the area that you're staying in, you might have to consider moving to another area in order to remain safe. But how does this work? What do you need to consider?

The Nature of Homesteading

Homesteading is the act of creating a life for yourself that is separate from the government and not reliant on it. In an emergency, there are several things you'll need to have in place: a supply of food that is stored, a supply of water, a method of transportation to get out of the city, and most importantly, a safe house in which you can stay. But what should this backup place look like?

Ideally, your shelter should be located away from the area you are currently staying. It should also be equipped with a number of items for survival: stored food, canned food, a large supply of fresh water, tools such as knives, guns, saws, axes, and first aid supplies. Your safe house can be located underground in a basement, but you will need to be willing to invest the money in having it built. This can be a costly business. Investing in structures known as bug-out bunkers can really save you a lot of hassle. These are prefabricated structures that can be easily put together and which contain all the necessary items you need in order to survive. Whatever method you choose to use for your backup shelter, always remember to have a backup plan. The essence of survival and prepping well is foresight.

Conclusion

In conclusion, the nature of being prepared lies in seeing what lies in the future and being ready for it. Those who fail to plan, plan to fail, as the old saying goes. In an increasingly unstable world, we need, more than ever, to show leadership and initiative in planning the course of our lives. This is what the prepping community is all about. Now you've read about how to survive and prepare wisely; there remains only one thing left to do, take the plunge and prepare. You now have the knowledge. But, without proper application, it means nothing. Whatever you want to do in life will only happen with your skill being applied to the situation.

References

6 Self-defense tips for urban survivalists. (2016, July 26). Urban Survival Site. https://urbansurvivalsite.com/6-self-defense-tips-urban-survivalists/

10 Simple survival shelters that will conquer the elements. (2018, November 21). Skilled Survival. https://www.skilledsurvival.com/survival-shelters/

10 Ways to find water to survive the wilderness. (2017). Know Prepare Survive. https://knowpreparesurvive.com/survival/10-ways-to-find-water/

54 item survival gear list. (2019, August 22). Skilled Survival. https://www.skilledsurvival.com/survival-gear-list/

Bachmann, D. (2021, January 22). *Staying warm in cold weather: Tips from an emergency medicine and survival expert.* Wexnermedical.osu.edu. https://wexnermedical.osu.edu/blog/staying-warm-in-cold-weather

Beginner's guide to (sane) prepping. (2020, September 14). The Prepared. https://theprepared.com/prepping-basics/guides/emergency-preparedness-checklist-prepping-beginners/

Burns: types, symptoms, and treatments. (2014). Healthline. https://www.healthline.com/health/burns#outlook

Charles, D. (2020, April 21). *Bushcraft: one of three ways to survive the Anthropocene.* Landscape News.

https://news.globallandscapesforum.org/44030/bushcraft-how-to-survive-the-anthropocene/

Davis, N. (2018, August 29). 8 *Self-defense moves every woman needs to know*. Healthline; Healthline Media. https://www.healthline.com/health/womens-health/self-defense-tips-escape#protection-alternatives

Dawson, D. (2015, February 20). *Self-defense techniques: be responsible for your safety*. Survival Mastery. https://survival-mastery.com/skills/defence/self-defense-techniques.html

Do you have a survival mentality? (n.d.) Mother Earth News. https://www.motherearthnews.com/nature-and-environment/do-you-have-a-survival-mentality

Durbin, L. (2013, October 9). *What's the difference between survival & bushcraft?* Low Impact. https://www.lowimpact.org/whats-the-difference-between-survival-bushcraft/

Edible wild plants: 19 wild plants you can eat to survive in the wild. (2010, October 6). The Art of Manliness. https://www.artofmanliness.com/articles/surviving-in-the-wild-19-common-edible-plants/

Emergency water for preppers part 2: purification. (2015, September 3). Backdoor Survival. https://www.backdoorsurvival.com/emergency-water-for-preppers-purification/

Finding food in the wilderness. (n.d.). Crisis Times. http://crisistimes.com/survival_food.php

Fishing weirs: how to build a primitive fish. (n.d.). Know Prepare Survive. https://knowpreparesurvive.com/survival/skills/fishing-weirs-build-primitive-fish-trap/

Here's what you need to know about escaping the mount in BJJ. (2018, April 11). Evolve Vacation. https://evolve-vacation.com/blog/heres-what-you-need-to-know-about-escaping-the-mount-in-bjj/

How to build a dugout shelter. (2020). The Survival Journal. https://thesurvivaljournal.com/dugout-shelter/

How to construct a full debris hut. (2018, June 9). Medium. https://medium.com/@Prepperadv/how-to-construct-a-full-debris-hut-step-by-step-c8f802eb7cf6

How to find drinkable water in the wild. (n.d.). Popular Science. https://www.popsci.com/story/diy/find-drinkable-water-wild/

How to find food in the wild: everything you need to know. (2018, September 17). Arbor Explorer. https://arborexplorer.com/how-to-find-food-in-the-wild/

How to get drinking water from plants and trees. (2018, April 9). Survivalist Knowledge. https://survivalistknowledge.com/how-to-get-drinking-water-from-plants-and-trees/

How to pick a suitable location for a survival shelter. (2014, October 3). Sunny Sports Blog. https://www.sunnysports.com/blog/pick-suitable-location-survival-shelter/

How to purify water in the wild. (2018, September 27). Uncharted Supply Company. https://unchartedsupplyco.com/blogs/news/purify-water-in-wild#_4.__

How to splint a finger. (n.d.). WikiHow. https://www.wikihow.com/Splint-a-Finger

How to stay warm in winter. (2019, February 16). Changing World. https://changingworldproject.com/how-to-stay-warm-in-winter/

Hunter, J. (2016, July 14). *The pyramid of wilderness survival food.* Primal Survivor. https://www.primalsurvivor.net/wilderness-survival-food/

Jeremy Anderberg. (2016, April 20). *How to find water in the wilderness.* https://www.artofmanliness.com/articles/how-to-find-water-in-the-wild/

Jones, B. (2018, August 3). *A beginner's guide to finding wild edible plants that won't kill you.* Popular Science. https://www.popsci.com/find-wild-edible-plants/

Jr, T. H. (2020, December 19). *Doomsday preppers stock up on luxury survival kits, emergency food supplies, and million-dollar bunkers.* CNBC. https://www.cnbc.com/2020/12/19/what-doomsday-preppers-stock-up-on.html

Knight, J. (n.d.). *Basics of wilderness survival shelters.* Alderleaf Wilderness College. https://www.wildernesscollege.com/wilderness-survival-shelters.html

MacWelch, T. (2018). *Consent form.* Outdoorlife.com. https://www.outdoorlife.com/survival-shelters-15-best-designs-wilderness-shelters/

MacWelch, T. (2019a, January 23). *3 tips to manage fear in a survival situation.* Outdoor Life. https://www.outdoorlife.com/survival-skills-potential-fear/

MacWelch, T. (2019b, January 23). *Overcome fear and panic in a survival situation.* Outdoor Life. https://www.outdoorlife.com/blogs/survivalist/2011/10/how-avoid-fear-and-panic/

MacWelch, T. (2019c, January 23). *Survival skills: how to build a fish funnel trap.* Outdoor Life. https://www.outdoorlife.com/blogs/survivalist/2013/05/surviv al-skills-how-build-fish-funnel-trap/

MacWelch, T. (2019d, April 24). *10 essential first-aid skills that every outdoors person should master.* Outdoor Life. https://www.outdoorlife.com/10-essential-first-aid-skills-that-every-outdoorsperson-should-master/

MacWelch, T. (2019e, October 21). *A guide to the 15 best survival traps of all time*. Outdoor Life. https://www.outdoorlife.com/how-build-trap-15-best-survival-traps/

MacWelch, T. (2020a, January 16). *9 natural shelters that will save your life.* Outdoor Life. https://www.outdoorlife.com/story/survival/natural-shelters-that-will-save-your-life/

MacWelch, T. (2020b, June 29). *Nine traits of the survival mindset that will keep you calm in regular life AND life-threatening situations.* The Budd Group. https://www.buddgroup.com/nine-traits-of-the-survival-mindset-that-will-keep-you-calm-in-regular-life-and-life-threatening-situations/

Macwelch, T. (2018). *Consent form.* Outdoor Life. https://www.outdoorlife.com/survival-skills-ways-to-purify-water/

McLean, S. (2017, November 27). *How to stay warm in the wilderness.* Survival Sullivan. https://www.survivalsullivan.com/stay-warm-wilderness/

Never starve: finding food all around you. (2019, April 11). American Outdoor Guide.

https://www.americanoutdoor.guide/how-to/never-starve-finding-food-all-around-you/

Reader's Digest Editors. (2019, January 10). *How to do CPR: 7 essential steps of CPR everyone should know.* Reader's Digest; Reader's Digest. https://www.readersdigest.ca/health/conditions/essential-cpr-steps/

REI Staff. (2018, April 2). *How to treat cuts, scrapes, and gouges in the Backcountry.* REI; REI. https://www.rei.com/learn/expert-advice/how-to-treat-cuts-scrapes-and-gouges-in-the-backcountry.html

SASI. (2014, February 11). *5 first aid survival skills you should learn.* Sasi Online. https://www.sasionline.org/survival/first-aid-survival-skills/

Spider shelter: surviving the wild outdoors. (2019, January 2). American Gun Association. https://blog.gunassociation.org/spider-shelter/

Stroud, L. (2019, April 18). *Finding water in the wilderness.* Scouting Magazine. https://scoutingmagazine.org/2019/04/finding-water-in-the-wilderness/

The rule of three - disaster survival. (n.d.). Know Prepare Survive. https://knowpreparesurvive.com/survival/rule-of-three/

Tilton, B. (2015, November 29). *How to build a survival shelter.* Scout Life Magazine. https://scoutlife.org/outdoors/3473/taking-shelter/

Torrey, T. (n.d.). *How to build a survival fire.* Instructables. Retrieved July 11, 2021, from https://www.instructables.com/How-to-Build-a-Survival-Fire/

Vartan, S. J. (2019, November 1). *Your climate change survival plan*. Medium. https://gen.medium.com/your-climate-change-survival-plan-69bd85ef12c8

Walter, J. (n.d.). *Winter survival: tips for staying warm in the wilderness*. Super Prepper. https://www.superprepper.com/staying-warm-in-a-winter-wilderness/#dangers

What is bushcraft? – bushcraft with David Willis. (n.d.). David Wilis. http://www.davidwillis.info/what-is-bushcraft/

What is bushcraft? bushcraft skills, tools, & how to learn. (2014, September 10). The Bug out Bag Guide. https://www.thebugoutbagguide.com/what-is-bushcraft-survival/#What_Are_Bushcraft_Skills

Wilderness survival: food procurement - animals for food. (n.d.). Wilderness Survival. https://www.wilderness-survival.net/food-1.php

Wilderness survival skills guide - finding and cooking food. (n.d.). The City Edition. https://www.thecityedition.com/2012/Wilderness_Survival3.html

Off-Grid Living

A Step-by-Step, Back to Basics Guide to Become
Completely Self-Sufficient In as Little as 30 Days
With the Most up-to-Date Information

Small Footprint Press

Introduction

Over the past year, there has been a sudden and powerful interest in leaving the cities and finding an independent life in the country. You probably feel those feelings, too. After all, you are reading this book. Well, you're not alone. There's been a massive exodus from some of the densest population centers in the United States. We have seen net population losses and places like New York, Nairobi, and Paris.

People are just sick of it. They're sick of the noise, the pollution, and the chaos.

People are leaving for places that have natural beauty. In Russia, people are leaving for country estates called *dachas*. In the U.K., people are leaving London and Edinburgh for the Scottish highlands. People are abandoning San Francisco and New York. We are watching a great migration from cities worldwide. After 2020, people don't want to feel confined anymore. People want to be able to walk outside freely. They don't want to feel dependent on strangers. They don't want to live every day feeling like they need permission.

It's no surprise then that so many people have been recently attracted to living off the grid. Living off the grid offers relief for many people who have been suffocating with those feelings and are ready to get out.

Cities are strange environments that we've created for ourselves. We could have made any kind of place to live, and for some reason, we chose to stack ourselves into tiny little apartments, 40 stories tall. We decided that this was worth paying $1,800 in rent every month.

New York had the good sense to set a bit of land aside and put some nature there, with Central Park. City planners had the foresight to know that if people were separated too much from nature, it would crush their spirits and make them feel crazy.

Now we are at a time where we don't even remember why we wanted to live like that. Lots of people are seeing it for the first time.

We Hear You

The people at Small Footprint Press know exactly what you're feeling. Our company was founded by people who felt the same way. That's why we wrote this book—there are people all over the world looking for some help.

Our mission is to empower people: to teach them to prepare themselves and their families for the challenges that come, so they can live their life securely, without fear.

Small Footprint Press is dedicated to a cause of a sustainable future, making the world a place where people not just survive but also thrive.

For that reason, we are happy to offer this book as a guide to help like-minded people live the best life they can. As part of our commitment to this cause, we donate proceeds from every website order to help protect our planet.

Something Better

Think of this book as a shopping catalog. You're building a new life, and you need to figure out all the pieces and how you're going to put it all together. The title of this book promises that you can live off-grid in 30 days. We absolutely stand by that. However, what that off-grid life looks like is entirely what you make it.

This is a primer to get you started; there is a lot more to learn. If you want chickens, you'll need to learn all you can about raising chickens. If you aren't going to raise chickens, then don't bother. Everyone has their personal needs, and we can't cover all of them in just one book.

In this book, we will cover a lot of the things that you know you don't know and many things that you don't know that you don't know. Get it?

Living off-grid simply means that you are living in a home that isn't connected to public infrastructure. That means you aren't connected to the electrical grid, the municipal water supply, sewage system, or telephone.

Some people enjoy living a very simple, primitive type of lifestyle that uses as little modern convenience as possible. Other people can live a completely normal modern lifestyle off the grid. You can find a place anywhere in between. If you want to live in a super minimalist, 18th-century lifestyle, that's fine. If you want to live a totally modern lifestyle off-grid, that's fine, too. It's just a matter of what you are looking for.

This book will cover a lot of topics, but it can't teach you everything you need to know. This one book can't train you to be a plumber, electrician, outdoorsman, carpenter, and farmer. What this book can and will do is give you a broad understanding of living off-grid, giving you the information and options to help you decide what's best for you and your family.

One topic that a lot of people might be interested in but we won't get into is prices. Prices are changing all the time. Wind power and solar technology are improving and becoming more popular, so we're seeing price decreases as it becomes more popular in the consumer market. Battery technology is getting better. There are also changes in the price of inflation and some recent political considerations that will affect the availability of imports.

For that reason, We're not going to tell you what things cost. By the time you read this, it's maybe totally different. You are going to want to do your own shopping and figure out those costs on your own. While some things are cheaper, and there's no reason to pay more for them, some things you get are exactly what you pay for. Suggesting you get the most expensive Gucci may not be appropriate and also saying you should get the cheapest one available might be a terrible idea.

Chapter 1:
Is off-Grid Living the Right Choice for You?

Living off-grid isn't for everyone.

There are some purists we'll say any connection to the grid means you weren't living off of the grid; we don't need to pay attention to them. There are levels of off-grid living. Between living in a tiny, cramped apartment in The Laurel on Manhattan's Upper East Side and living in a log home that's a 90-minute journey to the nearest grocery store, there is a wide spectrum. Imagine this book as a collection of tools and ideas with which you can build the life that you want.

Don't let that purest call you a phony. The words off-grid living are just words to describe a particular lifestyle. Don't hold on too tightly to the identity of it. This is about you living your best life and using your own self-reliance and will to create that life.

Living off-grid is all about self-reliance and self-determination. You have to be aware of nature and what it provides.

This isn't always easy, and it isn't for everyone, especially when just starting out. There are so many things to learn and so many trials that will challenge you along the way.

Living on your own, developing your self-reliance, and learning to take control of all of your own needs is not the easiest way to live a life but it is a rewarding one. It's one thing to work a job that pays you good money and make enough for a down payment on a home to live and maybe raise a family. There's another experience entirely of living in a home that you built.

What Is off-Grid Living?

It's very simple. Living off-grid means living a life disconnected from public and private utilities. That means you are disconnected from:

- the electrical grid.

- gas.

- municipal water supply and sewage.

- telephone lines.

It doesn't mean living without the things that those services provide. It means providing them for yourself.

Living off-grid does NOT mean:

- living in a medieval hut.

- abstaining from modern conveniences.

- cutting off contact from the outside world.

- growing a beard and living in a bunker, writing a weird manifesto.

You can do all those things if you want, but they don't have anything to do with off-grid living. There are many reasons why a person would choose to live off the grid. This is a lifestyle that attracts all kinds of people from all kinds of backgrounds. Ask yourself if any of these apply to you.

Green

Disconnecting from the grid means disconnecting from the energy system. Being able to produce your own energy from the sun, wind, and water is a way to reduce your impact on the environment. Perhaps you just want to separate yourself from the pollution of the cities.

Many people living off-grid have objections to the factory farming practices and would rather grow their own food than participate in the industrial food system. Plenty of people feel better knowing exactly where their food came from because they grew it themselves. They can grow what they like, and they always know it is free of GMOs and pesticides.

We're all aware of the electricity we spend in our homes. There's also the electricity that you don't see on your power bill every month. That electricity is factored into the price of every manufactured thing you own. Some of those items are manufactured abroad in places that have few environmental laws. Many of the things you own may have been built or manufactured using coal or oil energy, which are well-known pollutants. If you reduce your consumption by using the land, you can also reduce your dependence on the things that you don't agree with.

A self-sufficient lifestyle might help a person be more

conscientious about their own footprint and impact on global climate change. Many people have gotten into off-grid living as part of a movement of self-directed environmental personal responsibility. You probably can't change the world, but you can change yourself. If enough people do that, then we're all a lot better off.

Self-Reliance

There are plenty of people who simply like to be self-reliant. In the event of some terrible disaster, self-sufficiency will not be a problem for a person living off-grid. If the power goes out, they have power. If the water becomes a problem, they have water. If the cost of food spikes or there are shortages, that's not going to be a problem for a family who raises their own.

Overall, people just feel a sense of pride and accomplishment. Some people generally don't want to feel like they are a burden on others and that no other person is a burden on them. There's a certain kind of sense of security that you gain when you know that you don't need to rely on other people. If you only need to rely on yourself, and you are reliable, then you'll never be disappointed.

If you are the kind of person that wants to strike it out and make it on your own, and to build something that you can be proud of, homesteading might be something for you.

Privacy

Lots of people like privacy: They like quiet and solitude. If you are the kind of person who's inclined to walk around your house in the nude, you can do so without worrying about any neighbors peeking into the windows. In fact, you could probably just walk outside completely nude without any fear of phone calls to the police.

If you want to have guests over, play music, and have a bonfire and a good time outside, there is no one close enough to you to be bothered to complain. No one is going to come and knock on your door and tell you to keep down the noise.

Likewise, you don't have to deal with anybody else's noise. People in the city are accustomed to a lot of ambient noise. They have to hear traffic and cars honking their horns. The occasional car alarm goes off for no apparent reason at 1:00 a.m.; colicky babies screaming so loud that you can hear them through the walls of your apartment; and barking dogs, bravely protecting a homeowner from the dangerous pizza delivery guy who just arrived.

Being isolated can also isolate you from the problems in the city. If you live in a place with a lot of crime and violence, that tends to stay very local. Having a place relatively isolated is less likely to be targeted, so long as the owner takes the right precautions.

Investment

You don't have to be a hippie or a bearded mountain man to live off-grid. Sometimes, it just makes financial sense. A large off-grid project can have a big upfront cost, but over time, it can easily pay for itself from the savings on electric, water, gas, and food bills. Living off-grid may simply make sense for people trying to be thrifty.

If you buy or build a home in a very remote location, it may be way too expensive to get utilities out to your home. For completely practical reasons, connecting to the grid might just be unrealistic for you—this is more common than you might think. Homes built very high in the mountains or deep into the woods or country, without many neighbors, might decide that off-grid living is considerably less expensive than paying to have pipes and electrical lines built all the way to the grid to hook it up.

People who are investing in homes also often build off-grid sites to rent out to vacationers. Many people don't want to live in a remote place, far away from it all, but many people would love to vacation at a place like that. Making a remote and rustic off-grid location as a rental or vacation destination through one of the online hotel alternative websites could be a very remunerative enterprise.

Developing an off-grid home can require a good chunk of change. However, all of that money is an investment. Every addition you develop adds to the value of the land

and will come back to you when you sell—provided there is no terrible disaster, knock on wood.

There's been an increased interest in leaving the cities in the last year and people escaping into rural areas. One can probably expect that the value of the land is going to increase over time and not decrease. For that reason, having a self-sufficient and isolated spot that appeals to people trying to escape city life could be a valuable property to flip.

How Do I Know if off-Grid Living Is for Me?

Frankly, it might not be. Off-grid living is not for everybody. It takes a certain kind of personality to take on a project and commit to it. It takes a lot of self-reliance and eagerness to learn.

People have become very accustomed to convenience. Convenience is another word for time—as in saving time. Anything convenient saves time, but there is also a cost. Fast food is convenient. Ordering cheap things online is convenient. Sometimes, there are things more valuable than convenience. Also, the time that we are trying to save is just being wasted on other frivolous things.

These are some qualities that might determine if you are the kind of person who can do it. You don't need all of them, one is enough, but the more, the better.

Self-Starter

If you like projects, this is a great way to live. You will never run out of things to do. Many people make their home into their primary hobby. Are you the kind of person who is thinking about a good way to fix a squeaky garage door? Or the kind of person who builds a shed? If you're the kind of person who loves keeping busy and loves to work with their hands, you are in luck.

There are always new ideas you have for additions and for upgrades. Once your home is all put together, you'll start imagining other things you could build such as a sauna or a guest house. Once you get done with those, maybe you consider what it would take to build an artificial pond. If this sounds like you, keep reading.

Autodidact

That's not a type of dinosaur: An autodidact is a person who teaches themselves. You will need to learn a lot to live off-grid. If you don't like learning, this lifestyle will not work for you unless you learn. Learning is always going to be important.

Starting this life will make you a jack of all trades very quickly. To achieve absolute self-sufficiency, you will have to learn plumbing, electrical, farming, animal care, local law, and many other skills. Some people see that and want nothing to do with that. Others see a list like that and get excited.

This book is just the start of your off-grid education. There are many more resources that you will need to avail yourself of. Within a year, you'll know so much, you'll barely remember living another way.

If you like learning and are a very curious person who enjoys figuring things out and discovering new things, you will have plenty of opportunities. You will discover all the things you didn't know that you needed to know, and there are a lot.

Able to Follow Through on Commitments

You were meant to be someone who isn't a quitter. Depending on how you develop your land, there can be a large initial investment. It's totally possible to get started with $10,000, but depending on some factors, it could cost more. If you aren't serious about it, then you could easily waste a lot of time and money.

Pioneers and homesteaders of previous centuries did it with a lot less than we have available. Lucky for you, there are more tools and technologies available to you than they had.

By definition, you won't have an infrastructure around you that has been built up over a century by thousands of people who were financed by governments and corporations. You have to develop your own infrastructure from the bottom up. Over the long term, it can pay for itself.

This isn't like a month-long free trial at a gym or using a subscription service for a phone app. It's not the kind of thing you can half do by half measure. If you are a person who likes to finish what they start, and someone who doesn't rush into things, you have the right personality to live off-grid.

A Love for Nature

Last but not least, if you are looking to live off-grid somewhere that is far away from other people, you should be a person who genuinely loves nature. You are going to be surrounded by a lot of it.

Living off-grid means living in tandem with nature. You have to work cooperatively with it. Mother Nature decides when it rains, when the sun shines, and when the wind blows. While not everyone feels comfortable feeling at the mercy of nature, other people don't feel like they are at nature's mercy, but rather they are adapting to what nature prescribes. It's a very different attitude.

Maybe you really like living in a city where it's easy to find things that you need within a five-minute drive, and you don't like the unpredictability of nature. If you like gardening and animals, you'll have plenty of time with them. If you are someone who loves hiking, skiing, fishing, hunting, exploring, then this is where you want to be. Are you someone who loves campfires and loves to have their morning coffee on a porch overlooking a beautiful landscape? If so, you have come to the right place.

Healthy and Fit

People who have medical issues that require regular treatments and need to be close to the hospital or visit a clinic regularly are at greater risk if they live far away. Being off-grid doesn't mean that you can't be close to a hospital, but if you need a hospital to be close, be sure to factor that in. If you are planning on doing the work yourself, you should be healthy and able. People who are confined to wheelchairs might have a very rough time with it. However, if you're in a wheelchair and can build yourself your dream home, that would be very impressive and inspiring.

If you aren't strong or have good cardio, that problem will solve itself. You'll be chopping and carrying wood, building a fence, and all the other physical activities, plus a cellar without junk food—that will get you in a fitter state in no time.

Start Small

Living off the grid also doesn't have to be 100% complete on day one. Sometimes, the smartest way to start is to start small. Once you have a good piece of land that has all the features you need, you can get a trailer for relatively cheap to park there. That's a good place to start.

You can buy any water you need and bring it to your location. If you're ready now, just go and do it. Take it one step at a time. For most water systems, you'll need a pump. That means you'll need power. Power comes first.

You can start with a gas-powered generator until you can set up something more permanent. It won't be very long before you've set up your sustainable power system such as using solar power. Once that's up, you won't need a generator, then you'll be off the electrical grid.

You may have just put out some rain barrels to start with,

and that's fine. That'll help supplement any water that you are purchasing. When you get a well or more-developed method of getting clean water, you can stop buying it. Then, you'll be off the water grid.

You can rely on the grocery store when you begin and slowly phase that out as you build your garden and greenhouse, and build a coop to raise some chickens. Then you'll be self-sufficient for food.

There's no reason to start with the expectation that you will be completely self-sufficient on day one. Frankly, that's very unrealistic unless you can afford to have people come and completely design your project from the ground up before you even move in.

Start small and build out. Develop what you need to as you go.

As we say later on in this book multiple times, there is so much to learn. The best way to learn new things is to do them, so don't overwhelm yourself with tons of projects. Find one goal that you can accomplish and work on that. When it's done, continue to the next thing. If you come across any problems along the way, you'll figure those out and learn how to fix them, too. By the time you've moved to your next project, you'll already be an expert in whatever you just resolved.

As the subtitle of this book promises, you can live off-grid within 30 days, but you cannot build a gigantic off-grid compound with every luxury in 30 days. We don't know if it's possible to lay the foundation, build a house, and install plumbing and wiring in just 30 days. In some places, we don't think it's even possible to get a permit for construction within 30 days.

However, you can begin the moment that you have land. If you start small, you can be out there next month building toward something, so if you want to do it, sincerely, just go do it.

Mindset and Attitude

The off-grid mentality requires a balanced view of optimism and pessimism. You will need optimism to do the work and to believe in yourself that it can be done. It also needs pessimism because you will need to understand that things will go wrong—things that you cannot predict, and things that you should be able to anticipate. Your mantra should match that of the Scouts of America: Always be prepared. Just because your electricity is working doesn't mean that something won't happen to stop the electricity. Just because you have a car and you can leave doesn't mean that car will always work. Something happens to the car, and there is an emergency that requires you to get yourself or someone else to live with to a hospital, what is the plan B? If plan B fails, what is plan C?

The problem is that you can't anticipate, so you are going to have to figure that out. There are things you want to anticipate because you simply didn't know. You read this book and probably visited websites, read articles, and watched videos on the Internet, but there are things you know you don't know, like the weight of 14 ounces of mercury. There are also the things you don't know that you don't know. You can only learn these things when experience places them in front of you, and without any preparation for them, you will have to adapt and be creative.

Attitude and mindset are intangible things that you need to equip yourself with.

One thing to keep in mind is what it means to live isolated or far away from other people. If you are from an urban or suburban area, there are a lot of things that you take for granted. You have to understand what it means to be self-reliant in the context of living far away from people.

One thing to remember: If something goes wrong on your property, you are the first line of defense. If something that breaks down, you are the closest person to be able to fix it. You're not going to be able to rely on a landlord to come and have a look at it later the same day. If you need professional help, you're going to have to call them up, and they're going to have to drive out to you.

If you're a good distance away from town, you're going to want to have big trips. That means any kind of shopping you want to do, you should just choose a day and get everything done all at once—that means buying and bulk and getting lots of stuff. That means also thinking well in advance about what you will need, not just what you want for dinner tonight. You can't just go downstairs to the Bodega and pick up a sandwich. When you go to town, be sure to maximize your time and get plenty of supplies.

If you were injured, you might be a good distance from a hospital. For this reason, we strongly recommend that everyone get some kind of first aid training but especially if you live far away from the nearest emergency room. Living alone far away from other people can be risky. If you are not healthy or if you're not doing well, then you probably should have other people with you just in case. Something like a heart attack is a problem or much less lethal if you can expect an ambulance to arrive within seven minutes. However, if the nearest ambulance is 29 minutes away, you might be in for a lot of trouble.

This also means self-defense. When you live in an isolated area, the chances that someone is going to come and mug you, break into your house, or rob you are lower. However, if someone does try to come to your house with intentions, the police may be very far away. For that reason, you are going to be your own first and last line of defense. That could be surveillance cameras or security lights that detect motion. That could mean being armed. The point is, if it's just you out there, it may mean that nobody's coming to help.

Not having stores and other people available to you quickly means that you need to do what survivalists do. Any person who's into wilderness survival will tell you that you need multiple redundancies. That means if one of your pieces of equipment fails, you need to have a backup. When you are building your system, you are going to want to integrate multiple redundancies throughout it. That means multiple overlapping systems. If you can get electricity from two or more sources—if one of those sources goes down—you'll always have another one as a backup. If you can get water from more than one source, if you have a problem like a pump failing, then it won't be nearly as bad. This is especially true if you are totally relying on a car. If something goes wrong with your vehicle, and you need to leave the property in a hurry, you aren't going to have a ride-sharing driver just down the block, so you want to make sure that whatever vehicle you use is in tip-top condition, and don't leave anything to chance.

You have to think ahead more than you would living in a city. You have to think further in the future about living without your food and about possible problems with your water and power. You have to think about your own health and safety. When aid is always really close, you don't have to think about these things that much. When there's always a grocery store a couple miles away, you don't think about storing your food to last through the winter. A huge part of living an off the grid mindset is not preparing for the worst—not because it's likely but because something bad always happens eventually. Like the various Scouts of America say, always be prepared.

Kids

Going off-grid as a single person or with a spouse has certain natural advantages. You only need to care for the needs of two people. Going alone is dangerous because if something were to happen to you, no one is going to come looking for you. Someone is going to wonder why you didn't go back home.

Having children with you living off-grid has a lot of advantages and a lot of difficulties tied up with it. Well, children do have the power to contribute more and more as they grow older, and when they're very young, they consume more than they produce. A six-year-old can help out in small ways, but they need more help than they can give. Around the time a child is 10, and then in an off-road living environment, their contributions to the family and the consumption should be about breaking even. So, for the first decade of human life, they need more than they give. This means that adults need to produce more than they need to cover the distance. Adults produce their plus, and the rest goes to the children. This has been a fact that's been with us for the entirety of our species and before.

Plus, what is crucial in raising kids is education. Depending on how off the grid you are living in, you might not have realistic access to schools. You might have ideological disagreements with how the schools are handled because of religious or political differences. Maybe you just think that you can educate your children better than a state employee. Those things are true, you're going to need to homeschool your kids. Maybe you are perfectly happy with the education system, and you have an easy way for your children to go to school and come back. That's perfectly fine. You know what is best for your kids and family better than anyone else.

Chapter 2:
Location, Location, Location

Living off the grid also means living off the land. The place you select will have more impact on your off-grid lifestyle than any other factor.

Living off the grid is dealing with the uncertainty of nature.

Choosing a place is a tremendous commitment. If you are going to put all the work into making a place be sustaining, it needs to be the right place. You don't want to put a lot of time, money, and energy into something only to realize that it can't work for you. You need to really plan ahead. If you are close with your family, then being far apart from them might be a deal-breaker.

Location will determine a lot about the way you live. Your access to water, the soil, and other natural features will inform what energy and sources are available to you. The laws can be as important, if not more important, in determining how you get your water, how you get your electricity, how you heat and cool your home, and even what you eat. Make no mistake: Choosing where you live is going to be the most important decision, and there are a lot of factors that you need to balance.

How to Find the Perfect off-Grid Location

What is important to you will ultimately depend on you. No one can tell you better than you what your needs are and what kind of life you prefer. As we said in the introduction, this book is like a catalog of options that you can choose from.

Soil

If you are going to be doing any farming, the quality of the soil is going to be very important. You don't want to try to put in all the energy into starting a farm on land that won't give anything to yield. An easy way to determine if the land is good is just to simply look around. Are other people farming in this area? If they are, there's a very good chance that they know what they are doing and are using farmland.

This isn't a deal-breaker by any means. If the soil isn't great, you can buy soil at any home improvement store, you can add your own nitrogen, and use your compost to keep the mineral-rich earth. You can build a garden using raised garden beds for vegetables and herbs, using your own earth.

Not all locations are appropriate for certain kinds of farming. Depending on the season, soil, and climate, certain crops will be more amenable than others. You aren't likely to find very many tomato farmers in Alaska, for example.

Climate

Maybe that should go without saying but the climate is going to be crucial to how you organize your life. When living off-grid, you are dependent on nature to provide for you. Different climates have different advantages and disadvantages that you will need to weigh to make the life that you want.

Warmer climates are usually good for planting, however, you will have to deal with the problem of cooling yourself and any animals that you have. It's much harder to cool down than it is to warm up.

Likewise, wetter climates usually mean more water. They also mean humidity, which isn't great for humans, but it is nice for plants. Humidity also usually corresponds with plant growth. A lot of plants can block the wind and sun, which can make generating electricity more difficult if you're relying on solar and wind.

A nearby pond might be a great place to draw water and to raise fish. It might also be a potential breeding ground for mosquitoes.

Dry environments tend to be more comfortable. Arid areas also usually have more sun and wind, which is great for generating power. However, it may mean that getting water is more difficult or more expensive. Getting water is very important. Humans consume a lot of it, and your plants and animals will, too.

One very simple and important consideration is if you can even get onto your land. If your home is far away from the nearest road and you have lots of snowfall, you might be at risk of getting snowed in, and unlike other people who live in the city and subdivisions, there is no truck already on its way to plow the snow for you. Having a long road and heavy snow could mean you'll need a truck that you can mount a snowplow onto.

That's a lot of double-edged swords. There are advantages and there are drawbacks to everything. You have to seriously consider and weigh what is right for you.

Growing Season

Tied to climate and soil is the growing season. If you are going to be heavily reliant on producing your own food, you are going to want a longer and more productive season. You probably won't be doing that much growth during the winter. Historically, farmers plant in the spring, grow in the summer, harvest in the fall, and rely on their surplus during the winter.

Building a greenhouse can maximize productivity and extend the season if it is short. The more you grow and effectively store, the deeper you can fill your pantries and enjoy those supplies throughout winter. Luckily if you run out of food, you still have the option of driving to the local grocery store.

Water

The importance of water cannot be understated. When living in an arid place like parts of New Mexico and Australia, people are absolutely dependent on the water infrastructure. There is very little rainfall and very little access to natural water supplies.

Without water, you cannot drink; maintain plants or animals; take a shower, cook most foods; or wash your clothes or dishes. You absolutely need water, and getting water is your most important and most difficult task.

Your primary ways of getting water will come from a well, supplemented by rainfall. If you are lucky enough to have rivers or creeks that pass through your property or a pond—provided that there are no regulations against using that water—you can use those as well.

The Law

This is the least fun and interesting part of off-grid living, but it is very important. Making an error about the law can cost you a lot of money and trouble down the road. There's no use using common sense because laws often don't make sense. Don't assume that you are doing it right without checking first.

Between different states, there will be completely different regulations regarding building structures, digging wells, hunting, fishing, and every other thing that you can imagine. The number of laws is so vast and complex, we even have an entire profession to simply argue about what the laws actually are. They're called lawyers, and even they need to specialize in very specific areas of the law because there are so many.

If you aren't sure if something you were doing is legal or not, we strongly recommend that you don't just guess.

You need to investigate for yourself. Reach out to any local boards or administrative offices that handle that sort of thing—that means the DNR or the mayor's office. Even if they can't help you, they may be able to point you toward someone else who can.

Another useful resource is people who are also living the lifestyle already that you are working for. They have probably already experienced legal hiccups along the way, and if you can reach out to them, they can save you a lot of trouble. Look around on the Internet for forums and groups that are into off-grid living. If you can find others who live in a particular area, they might have answers to your questions.

Never ever buy land in a subdivision. Subdivisions are parcels that are pieces of land, part of a larger covenant agreement. If you have land that is attached to such an agreement, that means you are going to have a lot more rules that you need to follow. This is like having a homeowners' association and a bunch of neighbors who might have very strong opinions about what you do with your land. This isn't just true in the suburbs. You can also find properties like this in rural areas, so be sure to avoid this.

Keep in mind that agriculturally zoned land tends to be cheaper than residential or commercial land. If you can, buy agricultural land, and make sure it allows for ownership of livestock and farming. If you buy land that is zoned incorrectly, you might find that a lot of the things you want to do are not legal.

Believe it or not, some counties legally require you to hook up to city water. Whether or not you want to, you can be forced to pay for the installation of the pipes and hook up. This can cost you up to $10,000, or maybe more. This also goes for electricity. Some places legally require you to be on the grid. The whole point is to be off the grid, so don't go buying a place where you are not allowed to be off the grid.

There are also considerations of covenants and regulations about whether or not you can have a camper or trailer on your land and maybe rules about mineral rights or what requirements about a permanent foundation. You might find that a big part of choosing your land is about whether or not you can negotiate the obstacles set up by your state and local government.

Taxes and Exemptions

Tax laws are quite different from state to state. You may have to pay a rather large fee annually depending on the size and location of the land you are using. Depending on your budget, this cost could be an important part of your evaluation about where to homestead. Some places have no income tax; some places have low land taxes. These are things to take into account, depending on your finances.

There are certain tax write-offs that certain states offer that you can avail yourself of. A few states including Oregon and Utah offer tax deductions for using green energy on your property. Some states also offer tax breaks for those who use their land for farming. If you are building a new sizable grow operation, you might find that these rebates are worth your while.

Some states offer what's called the homestead exemption. That means that if you happen to go bankrupt and a certain portion of your land is filed as a homestead, then that portion of your land cannot be taken by creditors. The old traditional form of pharmacy went under during bad times, and workers would ultimately lose their homes—this is a law designed to protect people like that. Maybe you're not terribly concerned about going bankrupt and this is not a factor for you, but it is a nice thing to have all the same just in case.

Cost of Living

Money always matters. You may have a lot, or you may have a little. Your budget is your business, and budgeting might be a crucial factor for you.

Typically, the farther away you are from the city, the cheaper the land will be. People will pay a pretty penny to be close to a hospital or inside a good school district. The farther away you are from all of that, the less you need to spend. You might have to balance how close you want to be to civilization to how much you're willing to spend.

Sometimes, it can be hard to find banks that are willing to finance vacant land. Banks and mortgage companies like to sell you houses, not dirt. Often, the banks that will sell empty land charge more in terms of interest or down payments. One way around this is to work out a deal directly through owner financing. In this case, the bank operates as an intermediary where the lending agreement is directly between the current owner and the prospective buyer. The bank just gets a taste for mediating.

Everyone is living on different budgets and some places are simply more expensive than others. The prices of things are based on whatever the market will bear. Things that you want, such as natural beauty, are also going to be valuable to other people. This is one reason states like Geneva and Southern California are so expensive. Switzerland has access to a beautiful mountain range and nature. California has an entire coastline and beaches galore where you can search. Both have great weather.

Living near people with money costs money.

If you were living in a particularly remote area, things would just simply be more expensive because of the challenge of supplying areas. Areas in or around Alaska or island systems in places like Canada and Southeast Asia can be quite pricey because shipping to them is very expensive and difficult.

Natural Disasters

God forbid that you should experience any serious natural disaster. The odds that your home will be affected by one like that is usually pretty remote, but it shouldn't be ignored. You need to investigate if the area you're homesteading in is particularly vulnerable to flooding, tornadoes, or hurricanes. You need to think about these things ahead and have a plan ready so that you will know ahead of time and have a way to protect yourself.

Communication is important for this. If you live in tornado country, you definitely need access to the national weather service and a place to take shelter, such as a cellar. You want to be the last person to know there's a tornado, with no good way of getting away or taking shelter.

Homeschooling

For people who have kids, or who plan on having kids, school is very important. It matters in terms of quality but also accessibility.

If you are living very far away from schools, you might not have a bus that comes by your home. It might not be realistic to drive your kids to school and back, depending on the distance. Maybe you want to homeschool for ideological reasons.

Whatever the case may be, homeschooling might be important to you. Not all states are equally permissive about homeschooling. You will want to look into this and make sure that your state will allow it if that's important to you.

If you do decide to take the homeschooling route, now is a better time than ever. Homeschooling has come a long way over the last 20 years. There are all kinds of programs and lessons that can be bought online. There are many ways to meet with other parents and children to help them learn to socialize.

Access to Civilization

Some people can't safely live in an isolated area. If you have an illness that requires frequent visits to a doctor or hospital, you don't want to be too far.

Living off-grid does not mean you are living like a caveman or a 19th-century Canadian lumberjack. Being off of a utility grid does not mean being off of a social grid. You don't need to be socially isolated from other people. In fact, any psychologist will strongly recommend that you do not isolate yourself from other people. Just because you are living off the grid never means that you can't go into town to pick up supplies, and it doesn't mean that you can't go out to dinner or sports events.

The distance you are from your closest ER or grocery store might make a huge difference, in terms of driving time, gas, and emergency response. Being in a spot that is difficult for an ambulance to get to might be a deal-breaker.

Best States for off-Grid Living

These are 10 of the best states for living off the grid. This is not a top 10 list, and they aren't ranked from worst to best. Each of these places has its own strengths and weaknesses. Which is "best" depends on your needs and wants. No place is perfect for everyone, but there is a place that is perfect for you.

Look over this list and measure the pros and cons; from there, you can decide which place you feel is best.

North Carolina

"Nothing could be finer than to be in Carolina in the morning." North Carolina is a fantastic farm state, and there are many fellow homesteaders out there on account of their very friendly laws. Plus, since it's a great farming state with a long growing season and very beautiful agriculture, it also happens to be rather expensive. North Carolina is a nice state and you get what you pay for.

Pros

- gig farm state
- lots of homesteaders; ideal out west
- green rebate
- homestead declaration
- long grow season

Cons

- expensive land
- tight on homeschooling

Michigan

The wolverine state is not a bad choice at all. One of its most obvious and valuable features is that there is a ton of fresh water. The state is completely surrounded by enormous lakes, and on the interior are tons of smaller lakes. No one living in Michigan is too far away from a place to take a boat out to relax or to go fishing.

Michigan already has a pretty substantial homesteading community, and you are better off to find plenty of other like-minded people. The more northern in the state you decide to venture, the more open land there is.

One thing Michigan isn't running out of is fresh water. Michigan has all four seasons, although winters may seem a little long. The land is good for raising crops, but the season might be short. Maximize the season.

Michigan is also a great state for fishing. There are more lakes, and you can count plenty of salmon and trout that you can fish.

Michigan also has a large homesteading community. Having people who are also taking on the same project is always a great thing; making friends with others, you can learn a lot. In recent years, the price of living in Michigan has gone up, so take that into consideration.

Pros

- good soil
- short season
- lots of water for fishing
- many other homesteaders

Cons

- laws can be strict
- middle of road taxes
- complicated homeschooling laws

Tennessee

The beautiful state of Tennessee is one of the most underrated in the Union. It also happens to be the state that hosts The Great Appalachian Homesteading Conference. Like North Carolina, Tennessee is a state that is very friendly to homesteaders. While Idaho is getting a lot of love right now, the people of Tennessee should be glad that they haven't been discovered quite yet.

People living off the grid are generally more likely than a lot of people to get nailed with a panoply of natural disasters. Anyone living out there needs to take the proper precautions.

Pros

- mild climate with four seasons
- It's a beautiful state with great state and national parks.
- The cost of living is fairly low—it's about 10% less than the national average.
- There's good dirt for farming, especially in the west.
- plentiful water.
- Rural Homesteading Land Grant
- homestead exemption

Cons

- lots of natural disasters, including earthquakes, tornadoes, and floods.

Indiana

Indiana, like many other places on this list, is great for farming. They've got a good assortment of land and good growing season; they aren't hurting for water. At present, picking up rural land in Indiana may be tricky, so be sure to keep an eye out well in advance if you have any want on moving out there. One last thing, and we say this with all due respect, Indiana, besides homesteading, is a pretty boring state. If you like boring, that's great. If that's going to be a problem for you, maybe look around for other items on this list.

Pros

- mostly farmland
- longer growing season
- good homeschool
- good income tax

Cons

- might be difficult to get land
- high sales tax

Iowa

Iowa is of course a great farming state. They offer generous tax credits for farmers and homestead exemption, which is definitely a big help.

With no disrespect to the good people of Iowa, Iowa is not a very pretty state. It is mostly rolling planes filled with corn, wheat, and soybeans. It doesn't enjoy the beautiful forests of, say, Northern California and Iowa. It doesn't have the mountains of Tennessee and Colorado. It doesn't have beautiful bodies of water like Michigan or Florida. Iowa has many good qualities, but the natural aesthetic is not one of them.

Pros

- big farming state
- tax credits for farm
- homestead exemption
- low tax
- homeschool

Cons

- flooding
- Let's be honest. Iowa isn't very pretty. Sorry, Iowa.

Virginia

Virginia is a fantastic farming state and always has been. They have great rainfall, and they have access to the ocean. It's a very popular state for a good many reasons.

However, the problem with popular states is that they attract lots of people. Lots of people mean more expensive land, higher cost of living, and higher taxes. Unfortunately, that is a lot of the disadvantages of living in a city, except those disadvantages will follow you into the more isolated areas.

Pros

- There's great farming—Virginia is a farming state and always has been.

- good rainfall

- low property tax

- sell back electricity to power

- very popular

Cons

- expensive land

- high cost of living

- strict homeschooling

- disaster prone: hurricanes and flooding

Oregon

Once you get out of the Portland area, you will feel like you're in a completely different country. Oregon is a geologically beautiful state and very wet. Finding water in Oregon is as difficult as throwing a rock and waiting to hear it splash on something. You'll pay a hefty income tax if you make a lot of money, though.

Pros

- no sales tax

- lots of water

- few natural disasters

- green energy tax rebate

- rainy

Cons

- high income tax

Missouri

Missouri is very friendly to homesteads. They are very light with the regulation which is a major hurdle to overcome in more regulated states. In short, it's easier to do what you want with your property. The state is also geologically and vegetably diverse, and one part of the state will be quite different from another one.

Missouri gets a lot of rain. An average of about 40 inches per year, and it is legal to collect rainwater in barrels ("Average Annual Precipitation for Missouri," n.d.). Summers are very hot and can get very humid, but the winters are a little milder. By that, we mean a longer growing season but more need to keep your home cool.

Pros

- long season

- good rain

- good homeschool

- solar incentives

Cons

- rough winters

- high income tax

- natural disasters tornadoes flooding

Wyoming

The cowboy state is a strong option. It is the least populated state in the Union, and the land is pretty low cost. There is plenty of open space for solar and wind. However, sometimes too much of a good thing is a bad thing. Wyoming can have very powerful windstorms that are so strong that your roads are shut down for the safety of drivers. If you are in a location that is vulnerable to wind, you could find yourself in some difficulty. Also, your windmills might be great in most conditions, but powerful winds can sometimes be too much for them to handle.

Wyoming also happens to be a pretty dry state. Between the dryness and the strong winds, that means it also is rather vulnerable to fires. Wildfires are a fact of life in Wyoming.

Pros

- tons of open land

- low cost

- farming

- cheap

- no income tax

- relaxed homeschooling

- good for solar

- windy

Cons

- not much rain and wildfires

Idaho

Idaho might be America's best-kept secret. People who are already living there and know this don't want anyone else to know it, too. They like it the way it is and don't want to see it getting filled up with city people who are fleeing places like Los Angeles and Portland coming in and ruining it. As long as you don't tell anyone that you are from California, they will usually treat you well.

Pros

- Great farmland: A good percentage of the state are people who work in farming. There is a culture around it, and plenty of resources and help are available if you need it.

- Low cost of living: Things are just cheaper there, and they'll stay that way until people realize how great Idaho is.

- Green energy benefits: At the time that this book is being written, Idaho offers tax benefits for people who use green energy.

- Homeschool-friendly options: If you want to homeschool your kids, Idaho won't get in your way.

Cons

- high taxes
- natural disasters

A Few Great Spots Outside of the U.S.

The U.S. is great for homesteading and off-grid living, but it is far from the only country you can go to. There are very innovative and adventurous homesteading communities all over the world. Here are a few of our favorites.

Raoul Island, New Zealand

As anyone who has watched *The Lord of the Rings* movies knows, New Zealand is one of the most beautiful countries on Earth. Raoul Island is a small island with a small population. Almost everyone there lives completely or partially off-grid. The climate is fantastic and you can live in paradise.

Pros

- Off-grid community already there
- Excellent climate
- Unbelievable scenery
- Great fishing

Cons

- Outside supplies need to be shipped in
- Not cheap

Lasqueti Island, Canada

Located in Vancouver, British Columbia, Lasqueti Island is the home to about 400 people in an off-grid community. If you've never been, Vancouver Island is absolutely gorgeous and has everything you need. Vancouver Island has several privately owned islands, so if you are looking to relocate to an excellent off-grid location, you should probably check them out. They are happy to see any visitors who want to check the place out.

Pros

- Beautiful environment
- Great access to fresh water
- Access to fish
- A community that are already pros

Cons

- It can be difficult to get a work permit in Canada
- It's an island and the only way to leave is by boat or ferry

Khula Dharma, South Africa

Khula Dhamma is an "eco-village," an experiment in green living. People live in updated versions of traditional African huts. Straw and clay make for excellent insulation against Africa's hot climate. This community is self-reliant. They produce their own food, electricity, and water.

Pros

- Anyone looking to be green will love this place
- Very knowledgeable bunch of people
- Inexpensive

Cons

- Perhaps too rustic for some people
- There is an application process to join the community
- Hot

Off-Grid Homes

Living in a home that you built creates a certain intimacy with your environment that's difficult to put into words. People who have done it understand this even if they've never tried to articulate it before.

Imagine you live in a place where every single board is there because you put that board there. Every single nail was hammered into place with your own hands. You know every inch of electrical systems. All the pipes are exactly where you chose to put them. You know how all of these systems work because you couldn't have put them there without knowing it. Better yet, inside of this house are memories of the trials, difficulties, and problems that came along while you were building the home. Each of those memories is a fond one because it is the memory of a challenge that you overcame.

The self-made home contains the story of the conquest over challenges and the pride of doing it yourself. You will live inside of a shrine of your own accomplishments. It's not easy to put a price on that.

There are stories of people who are offered large amounts of money to sell their homes to developers who aren't interested in the home itself but are interested in the land for a larger project. You'll often hear these stories of people who are in their later years, refusing to sell at any price. They're living in a home they built themselves or built by their parents or their spouse. It's one thing to live in a place for a long time and call it home. It's another thing to create a home.

Fair Warning

Before doing any work on your property, it is extremely important that you investigate the laws in your state or accounting to make sure you aren't accidentally breaking any. Every place is different, and there's no reliable way to know what you can and cannot do by just using your own common sense. You may need to purchase permits; you may need to use licensed contractors. We would recommend that you reach out to your local government. Call them, or even better, show up in person and ask them directly.

In one example that we know of personally, a person dug their own well on a property. There was nothing illegal about that, however, for someone to get a bank loan to purchase the property, they needed it to be inspected.

During that inspection, they saw that the well was not installed by a person with the state certification. The banks would not loan money to anyone to purchase the property without the certification by the well digger. The owner would have to destroy the well and replace it with another one or find a person who was willing to purchase the property upfront in cash. Needless to say, it was a huge disaster.

Making this mistake can mean that you waste your money with whatever development that you're putting into it; you'll also have to waste money to tear down whatever development you made on the property, and then waste even more money doing it the prescribed way. If you accidentally violate an ordinance, you will be fined over and over until the issue is settled. If you can't settle it, the state could take your land from you to pay off the debts from the fines that you can't pay.

Do not make the mistake of assuming you know what the rules are. Unless you are an expert and have a career developing in that particular area, you need to double-check everything.

Cabin or House

It's the most obvious living situation, and that's why it's the first one. This is going to be the option that most people will go with if they plan on staying on the property long term. Houses are not easy projects, as any homeowner will tell you. When you are adding on the additional challenges of off-grid living, that then means there will be a few other considerations to be mindful of.

Building a cabin has a lot of rewards, though. If you have a family, then you are going to need a place big enough for all of them. If you are laying down roots and really trying to start a life somewhere, this is a good choice. If you are simply trying to improve the land so that you can rent out your property for Airbnb, small rentals, or to eventually sell, building a cabin is the sensible choice.

If you have a big family and need a house, build a house. If it's just you, and you are starting small as we recommended at the start of this book, don't feel like you need to jump into this right away. If you don't need a house, don't get one until you do.

In some rare cases, you might be renovating an older place and retrofitting it to work off-grid. This can be harder than just building a new place from scratch. A lot of off-grid resources are most efficient when they are integrated with the house. It's difficult to build something like a radiant heat floor if the floor is already built. Some old houses might be great candidates for renovation, but I'd recommend against it unless you really know what you are doing.

For the majority of you, you will pay to have a house built, or you will build some of it yourself and hire contractors for other parts. You may not feel qualified to lay a foundation or to install an electrical system. If you are a DIY kind of person and you have the time to do the work yourself, it can be a great experience. If you are an experienced contractor, then you can just continue to the next chapter because you probably already know exactly what you're going to build.

Yurt

For the homesteader who wants to live a more old-fashioned and primitive type of lifestyle, there's always a yurt. Not everyone wants to keep all the luxuries and indulgences of modern civilization—many people would like to get away from those things. These are small, one-room buildings. Some people will build several on their property, so everyone living on the property has their own.

These can be very nice and well done. They are very affordable, cozy, and charming. They're not always great if you would like a lot of privacy from other people you share the property with. They are also a project that is doable for the layperson. A house is a lot, but a nice yurt is within the reach of someone who isn't a pro but would like to make their own home.

Vehicle

Some people like to live in a vehicle. This is a very neat option if you don't like to stay around in one place for very long. If you are in a position in life where you like to travel, you can bring a lot of your home with you. Maybe your land is where you call home, but you move around enough that it just makes sense to live in a home with wheels and an engine. You can have a power system and water system waiting for you when you come home.

Living in a vehicle doesn't always mean living in a camper. There is a large community that likes to refurbish and retrofit large vehicles to live in them. This could just mean something as small as a van, but people have gone as far as refurbishing former ambulances with excellent suspension for traversing difficult mountainous areas. Some people have fixed up vehicles that are out of service or retired school buses and rebuilt them into serviceable homes. There's a tremendous amount of interest in creativity in this lifestyle. Do an Internet search for "van life" and you'll see how popular this trend is, especially with young people.

Shipping Container

It's more common than you may realize, but people have built homes and even larger compounds out of shipping containers—those are those large rectangular boxes made of corrugated steel that they used to ship goods across the ocean.

If you search on the Internet for many of these things, you might be very impressed with what you find. People have designed remarkably modern and interesting homes by stacking containers and welding them together. They look a lot nicer than we are describing them, and obviously, a lot of work is put into them to achieve that. There's also been a recent surplus of shipping containers after the COVID-19 pandemic, so getting them now is cheaper than ever.

One technique is to bury the container mostly with dirt with one end of it open. This essentially looks like a hill with a door in the side of it, like a hobbit's home you would see in *The Lord of the Rings*. The drawback here is that you will need a heavy machine to move that much dirt, and you will not have any windows because it is essentially underground. On the plus side, it feels kind of cool, and it has fantastic insulation. When you are mostly underground, you are essentially using a geothermal conditioning system that keeps your home warmer in the winter and colder in the summer.

Micro Home aka Tiny House

Micro homes are a strange and adorable trend. These are exactly what they sound like: They are super small and very efficiently organized—and very cheap—homes. You can buy a lot of them almost completely put together. Think of them as recreational vehicles without wheels and much nicer overall.

People have also taken tiny houses and built tiny house communities. They are small enough that they can be taken to even tiny plots of land relatively easily. People who live in these are often off-grid and rely on a lot of solar and wind power and rainwater. This is a really great option for someone young and single. This is definitely not an option for people with families who need space. If you can comfortably fit your life inside of a New York apartment, then you can live in a tiny house.

Chapter 3:
Off-Grid Water System

According to the United States Environmental Protection Agency (EPA), the average American family uses 300 gallons of water a day. That isn't a typo. That's 300. 70% of that water is used inside the home and breaks down as follows ("How We Use Water," 2018):

- 24% toilet
- 20% shower
- 19% faucet
- 17% clothes washing
- 12% leaks
- 8% other

The other 30% is used outdoors for washing cars and watering lawns. Needless to say, we use a lot of water.

That number can be cut down dramatically if you are responsible and conscientious, but even if you can manage to cut that number in half, you still need a lot of water.

At a bare minimum, you're going to want 500 gallons of water on hand at any one time. That's water that's already been pumped or collected and stored in a cistern or tank. If you can get more than 1,000 gallons and safely store them, that will make your life much easier. Storing water is crucial for survival, and it can also be important for other systems that your house uses, such as heating.

Cleaning

Before we even get started on collecting water, we must talk about getting clean water.

Clean water is a serious problem in many parts of the world. In the developing world, poor access to water, or water contamination, is a tragedy. For most of human history, finding a reliable source of clean drinking water was very difficult and crucial. This is why ancient cities were always built on rivers for fresh water.

Water straight out of the ground or a pond is not going to be clean. It will have mud, clay, and a lot of other gross stuff you don't want to drink. Wherever you get your water from, you are going to need to include a filtration system—that includes rainwater. Water captured in barrels still probably touched a roof and gutter to be collected. And still water in a barrel is a breeding ground if it isn't treated.

The biggest risk is any form of contamination by microorganisms. If you ingest these, they can seriously mess up your guts. Water can also be contaminated by gas or contaminants that are leaking into the soil.

Do not drink unfiltered water. Water contains all kinds of microscopic organisms that will seriously harm you and potentially kill you.

Simply boiling water kills many different types of contaminants but not all. Most viruses of the bacteria won't survive as they boil. Others can survive it and can only be killed with a very high temperature, usually requiring a pressure cooker. Boiling may be a good enough solution for a short-term survival situation, but boiling water in a pressure cooker is not a good long-term system.

Modern filters are so tight that the gaps in the mesh are measured in fractions of a micrometer. This means most microscopic particulates and organisms cannot get through it. It's also a great way of moving any kind of junk in your water. They usually contain a mix of ceramic and carbon, which are the same thing that they use in the water filters that attach to your sink or use in a pitcher. Filters will need to be replaced, periodically. Consult the instructions of any filter you use.

For your rain barrels, you might want to use tablets. Water purifying tablets kill most biological invaders. Tablets usually use iodine, chlorine, or sodium, so you need to be careful not to overtreat the water. You do not want to be consuming too much of the stuff that cleans the water. Purifying tablets also can't remove any harmful particulates such as heavy metals.

Ultraviolet light can purify water by killing microbes' ability to produce. Light-treated water needs to be used shortly after cleaning or stored in a lightproof location. Normal exposure to light can recontaminate the water.

If you have no access to water, then you have probably chosen a bad place to live. If for some reason you find yourself in a position where you only have access to saltwater, solar-powered desalination is an option.

In short, to get safe water, you are going to have one or more solutions to handle both biological and nonorganic junk.

Rain

Rain is free, easy, and clean. It falls from the sky, and all you have to do is catch it before the earth drinks it. Setting up a series of rain barrels is the simplest way to do this.

You want to use any large surface area as a way to collect. Easy examples are the roof of your home and solar panels. The water can be caught using gutters and delivered into barrels. Just leaving a bunch of barrels out in the yard is not going to be very effective if you want to maximize the space to capture.

As we mentioned earlier in this chapter, barrel water needs to be treated. You absolutely do not want algae or mosquitoes finding a home inside of it.

Rainwater is great but it will not be enough for you. If you live in a very rainy environment and it's just you, maybe you can get away with it—probably not, though. For most people, especially those with children, rain barrels are a very important part of the water system, but they are not enough themselves. Rain barrels are supplemental. They won't be the most important water source.

If you can, have the rainwater diverge directly into one of your main tanks. If you can't do that, you can add the water directly to the tank manually if you don't mind a little bit of heavy lifting. Rainwater can also just be used as a gravity shower.

In the winter, your rainwater is now snow water. If you heat it up, it will serve the same function. It's also much easier to collect because it's all over the place, and you can just scoop it up.

Believe it or not, harvesting rainwater is actually illegal in some places. Make sure you won't get a fine for catching the water from the sky.

Wells

For your main water source, digging a well is by far your best bet. Rain is fine if there's a supplement. Creeks and ponds might not be available or legal to take from. Delivery is fine temporarily, but it's not a permanent solution. If you're going to be living somewhere, you want a permanent, stable, and reliable source of water—that means a well.

Shallow Well or Pump Well?

If there is water high enough, you may be lucky in that you can dig a shallow well. Basically, what you do is get an excavator to dig out a big hole in the ground, about 10 feet in diameter and around 18 or 20 feet in depth. If you're finding water at that depth, you are in luck. I'll keep saying it: Check your laws. Some pumps that go deeper than a precise number of feet are regulated. Yes, the laws are that finicky.

Once you have a hole, you can install the pipe, valve, and pump, and run the pipe up over the top. Then, fill in the rest with gravel, then cover with dirt.

If you are feeling really rustic; you need water now but don't have electricity yet; or if you want a second, minor well, you can always use a lever hand pump—very old-fashioned but very effective for small amounts of water. Not a great way to get water for your whole house, but it's great as an intermediary step or a supplementary system.

Deep Well

One thing that's been a problem with settling new land is finding locations to dig a well. It wasn't that long ago that con artists were making money using dowsing rods, wandering between the town, and promising they could detect places that were good for a well. Then he'd take their money and disappear before the people who hired them were able to realize their mistake.

Any piece of land that you want to dig a well on, you should investigate ahead of time. It would be a good idea to reach out and talk to the neighbors first. See if anyone else nearby has dug their own well. If none of them have, you might be able to speak with folks in the city about any records they have of natural resources. If you are going to need a well, you should use land where you are likely to find water.

Digging a well blind is extremely risky. If there are no other wells nearby and you don't have good information on the water table, you are firing blind.

You may be able to take a relatively shallow well with just an auger and get very lucky. However, in some places, you need to dig and install pipes that are hundreds of feet down. Every single one of those feet costs a lot of money. Maybe you get lucky and you find water 40 feet down. Maybe you don't get lucky and drill down 300 feet and still find nothing. The people who dig the well get paid whether they find water or not.

A well is probably your best source of water, but if you are not careful, you can end up spending a tremendous amount of money with no benefit, so be very careful.

Digging a well may be one of the most expensive projects to get your off-grid home up and running. However, on the plus side, adding a well will greatly raise the property value. As long as you did it with a company following all the rules and licenses, the value added to the land should pay for itself if you ever decide to sell.

Springs, Rivers, and Creeks

If you find a river or creek on your land, you may feel like you have an excellent supply of water. We hate to break it to you, but a lot of states do not allow you to draw water out of creeks, rivers, and ponds crossing through your land. This is doubly true out west. Where water is especially scarce, they have appropriative water rights. That makes it illegal to draw water from a naturally occurring source.

That creak, stream, or river you have somewhere potentially crosses through somebody else's lawn on its destination to some other larger body of water. It would be seriously uncool to interfere with that stream as across as someone else's land. That's why you can't just build a dam and divert the water in another direction. That messes with someone else's property.

If you were grabbing some 100 gallons a year, you might not get caught, but we cannot recommend that you break state law to get water when there are other ways to do it. You may just have to enjoy the calming and serene bliss of the water, but tragically, you won't be able to take a shower with it.

Delivery and Pickup

In survival training, they will teach you that you can go three hours without shelter, three days without water, and three weeks without food. We need to upend that rule a little bit on our priorities. To get water, we need to pump. To get a pump working, we'll need electricity, so electricity is actually more important than water.

If you're developing an area with a hill, you can make things easier for your pump by putting water cisterns on top of the hill and running a line to your house, trenching it, and burying it underground. Natural gravity will give you natural water pressure without requiring any extra electricity.

When you first start your off-grid home, it may be a while before you can get access to your own water. You may be reliant on water from outside. If you have tanks set up and buried, with valves and pumps installed, and pipes going to your home, you can hire a truck to deliver water and fill up your tanks. If not, then you can go to the store and pick up as much as you need and drive it back.

This is not a good long-term solution to your water problems. This is just costing you gasoline and time, plus the water is more expensive than if you were on the grid. You can rely on this kind of water supply for a short time while you are getting your permanent water system fully operational. Also, if there's some kind of problem down the road and you need to do repair on your system or something gets funky, you can get the water delivered if it's the last resort.

We're only including it in this book because realistically you will be using delivered water for a short period at the start of your off-grid homesteading.

Storage

Water needs to be stored. You won't be pumping water every time you turn on a faucet. Water is pumped and stored in tanks as needed. Your indoor water is drawn from the tanks. The bigger the tanks, the more water you have at the ready. You want large volumes of it ready to go.

Like everything else, if you want to be prepared and have more than you need, get it now because you might need it later.

Tanks and cisterns should be stored underground. After just a few feet into the earth, the ground is cool but not frozen. This is important because in the summer, the place under the ground will not begin cooking near water and making it 90 degrees, and in the winter, it won't freeze or burst and become impossible to use.

Any kind of pump system will also need to be underground including the valve. Just like the water, you do not want the mechanics of getting the water out of your pump to freeze—that would be a serious disaster. How much water you'll need and how big your tank is will depend on your personal needs, but we always recommend getting more than you need just to be safe.

Water collected from rain can always be added to your tanks to top them off and give your pump a break.

Chapter 4:
Generating off-Grid Power

Power Sources and Saving

Renewable energy has come a long way, but it isn't a fully mature technology. Like everything in life, there are trade-offs. They have pros and they have cons.

Solar and wind power can generate a tremendous amount of energy when the sun and wind are at their peak. This is great except for one big problem: They create more energy than is needed. The surplus energy can't be stored safely because battery technology hasn't been able to keep pace. When the solar panels aren't catching the sun or when the wind isn't blowing, they produce nothing. We need energy when we need it, not just when nature provides it.

On a municipal scale, this means that green energy still has to be supplemented with other energy, be it nuclear or coal. On a small scale, you can be flexible enough to make it work. Living off-grid means living on an electrical budget. You're going to want to get a good estimate of how much energy you need. If you can get an estimate for how much energy you are using now, you can get a sense of how much energy production you're going to need on your off-grid home.

1,000–1,500W is probably enough juice for your needs, but everyone's needs are different.

The power source you use will depend on your environment. The more you can mix your energy sources, the better. If one isn't generating, another one might be able to make up the difference. Diversity of energy is reliable energy.

Naturally produced energy is about living on nature's schedule. When it offers you wind or sun, you take it while you can get it. If you are using naturally produced power from wind and solar energy, you are living on an electrical budget. You have to regulate your own energy use because you can just use as much as you want and pay a bill for it later.

One way of handling this is by using the power when you have the power. This is called "opportunity usage" and is a very effective way to maximize your power. Schedule all of your heavy electrical activities for when the sun is up and the wind is blowing, and there will be no wasted energy. If you have a washing machine and dryer, and you have a sunny day, that would be an excellent time to do your laundry.

Solar

Solar energy is cheaper and more available now than it has ever been before. It's so common that it's no longer unusual to see solar arrays attached to the roofs of someone's home. Solar panels are made of crystalline silicon wafers. Contact with sunlight causes electrons to move about inside of them, and this flow of electrons is what generates an electrical current.

Big solar farms optimize the energy to drop in the sun by turning the panels automatically to always face the sun and have the optimal angle with more maximum coverage of the surface area of the panels. This is exactly how sunflowers operate—they always move to face the sun so they can get as much sunlight as possible.

Not all solar panels are equal. Some people simply lay them flat on the ground—that is the least effective way of catching the sun. It'll be great and high noon during the summer when the sun is directly above it, but it will be increasingly useless as the sun goes down.

Higher-end models can do what those major industrial solar panels do, and follow the sun. They are definitely more expensive, but they may be worth the initial investment if you can get more juice out of them and optimize your array.

Most people find that installing panels on the roof of the home is the smartest option depending on the way that they face the sun. Many people set up arrays on towers about the property, in areas where there isn't any shade or trees blocking. Very often the best place to put your solar array is in the garden for the same reasons. It's an open space with lots of sunshine.

You can't make a solar panel system without some electrical skills. If you know something about wiring up an electrical system, or you are willing to learn, you can do it yourself. However, it can be risky if you are inexperienced. Faulty craftsmanship can damage some of the systems and cost you money and time.

Building your own system takes planning and research, and, as we say many times in this book, always be sure to check out your local regulations. Some places require permits or official qualifications.

Solar panels also need to be weatherproofed. After they are put up and jointed together, they need to be sealed so that water and moisture do not get into them. Make sure that any panels that you purchase are from a reputable supplier and manufacturer. Getting cheap panels from an untrustworthy supplier could result in a fire. Look around. If something seems so cheap that it's too good to be true, it is. Safety first.

You can build solar panels from scratch out of individual solar cells if you like. It's not too difficult. You start by creating a backing for the panel. You can use a wooden board, and you will need to drill holes and then at the right place so that wires from each cell can pass through the back. They are then wired together using a soldering iron. They should be attached to your backing individually so that they can be removed individually. If a single solar cell is damaged, it should be relatively easy to remove the single damaged cell and replace it without having to replace the entire thing.

A solar panel by itself doesn't do anything without an electrical system. You need to pair your panels with an inverter to turn the direct current (DC) into an alternating current (AC). Nearly everything you use requires AC power. Running DC into that stuff will not work.

Before you even begin designing your system, you should probably get a sense of how much power you will need. Look at your current electrical bill, and you might be able to get an estimate of how much juice you are using. Then, look at weather reports to see how many days of sunshine you get on average in the area that you are building. With a little bit of math, you should be able to get a sense of what the scope of your solar system needs to look like.

For beginners, we recommend that you purchase solar panel kits that come with all the instructions included and all of the tools necessary to build your solar system. Good kits also include racking and a means of mounting your system. If you want to do it yourself but don't really know how, these kits are definitely a wonderful option.

Wrecking refers to installing it to either the ground or onto the roof. If you are using an RV, then you will need to mount it on that. Whichever method you use, these must be very secure; you don't want them falling off or getting blown away by gusty wind. It might be a good idea to get your solar panels from the same place you get your racking supplies to guarantee that they will fit together. Even though some companies promise compatibility, these things can sometimes be like blue jeans. The size on the label says one thing, but when you actually try it on you find it isn't quite what was promised.

Working with a professional who is a trained electrician with expertise in solar panel installation will be likely your best bet. They know all the laws and regulations, they are experts in their field, and they are probably going to get it right the first time. If you are a DIY person who knows a little bit of that electricity and is willing to learn a lot more, this can be a great project for you to take on yourself. If you don't feel up to it, letting a professional deal with it is a good call.

For those living in places like the Pacific Northwest of America or Scotland, catching the sun won't be reliable. You can keep adding panels, but the better choice is to add other energy sources.

Wind

If you live out in the open in a windy place like Argentina, Perth, or Wyoming, the wind is a great option. If you live deep in the woods, you might not get enough wind to make it worth your while. Trees do a great job of breaking up the wind and giving you shelter from hurricanes and dangerously forceful winds. Unfortunately, it also means you can't get wind power.

Wind turbines are commercially available, but they aren't cheap. Some can generate as much as 3,000W—emphasis on CAN. Like solar power, just because the box says it can generate a large wattage doesn't mean that it will. Nature makes that decision.

A lot of areas do not like the look of windmills, and regulate them. Like everything else, check the laws to make sure you're allowed to have them. Windmills also need to be mounted on polls. Usually, higher is better, as there is less obstruction from your buildings, hills, and trees. Around 20 feet should do the trick in most cases.

Geothermal

Geothermal is a very cool option with one major drawback: Getting it up and running can be very pricey.

Geothermal energy is not actually producing electrical power. It just makes heating and cooling easier and more efficient.

Geothermal works by drilling a deep hole in the earth and running water through it. The deeper into the earth you go, the less affected it is by the temperatures on the surface. In effect, the temperature is stable.

When it is ferociously hot outside, the temperature deep in the earth is cooler. When it is intensely cold outside, the temperature in the earth is warmer.

The more you want to change the temperature, the more energy you need. It takes more heat to make ice into a gas than it does to turn liquid water into a gas.

Geothermal works by splitting that amount of energy by meeting your energy need halfway. If you need to cool things down, the geothermal temperature gets you halfway from hot to cold. If you need it warmer, then it's the same thing.

It is very simple, practical, and most importantly, reliable.

This is highly recommended. It doesn't provide electricity, but it makes your electrical systems much more efficient for heating and cooling your home and water.

Micro-Hydro

This is a very interesting option if your spot has running water. Unlike solar and wind, a moving river or creek is always moving. Depending on the time of year, you'll get more or less power, but it's always there for you if you need it.

Reach out to the Geological Survey or Department of Agriculture. They may have data on the speed and force of the water moving through your property. If it isn't strong enough, hydropower might not be worth your time. If your water source does produce enough force, like every other improvement on your land, you should contact whatever local department is in charge of energy or natural resources and ask them about the rules for diverting water.

If you have a green light for those two items, you'll need yourself a generator, turbine, and piping. Consider yourself lucky because this is not an option that is available to most people living off the grid.

Gas-Powered Generator

A generator isn't anyone's first choice, but it's important to include. It uses gasoline—which is expensive and a pollutant—it's loud, and it smells bad. That said, you're going to want one.

You may need a generator to get by while you are getting yourself set up. Until your other power sources are up and running, you will need something.

It's important to have a generator in case of emergencies. Even if you seldom need it, you'll be very happy to have it when you do. As we discussed earlier, several overlapping redundancies are crucial. You'll want a generator just in case. If you accidentally leave your keys in your truck overnight and drain your car battery, you will be very grateful to have a generator.

Important note: Gasoline goes bad. Gas is perishable. It has a shorter life span than you might realize. If you have a spare plastic tank of gas, you will need to change it out periodically. Pure gas that is properly stored can last six months. Gas blended with ethanol lasts three months, so keep this in mind. You don't want to fill a tank with bad gas.

There are options for petroleum-based stabilizers to add to gas, which will extend its life to one to three years.

If your gas looks too dark or you see any sludge in it, it is old, and you can't use it. Putting old or contaminated gas can ruin the machine you're trying to power.

Storage

Energy storage is going to be necessary because the wind won't always be blowing, and the sun won't always be shining. To store the energy, we have two main options.

The obvious answer is batteries. There are lots of options, and not all batteries are created equal. You can get heavy acid batteries, the kind that is used in golf carts. Those are a fine option and relatively cheap, although they are heavy and filled with acid, and you do not want to tip them over because they are full of liquid. You can also find lithium batteries, the same type used in your cell phones. These are cheaper but also more expensive and often have less capacity.

Obviously, you're going to need an electrical system to build these batteries and then to pull power from them when needed into any other electricity you are using in the home.

Battery storage is measured in ampere hours. That means a 100-ampere hour battery will give you 100 amps for one hour . . . sort of. Batteries also have a natural discharge rate. This is called Peukert's law, which complicates the math a little. Batteries have different discharge rates that will also affect how much juice you get out of them. People who know a lot about this will check batteries for Peukert exponents.

The discharge rate can also be affected like the temperature and how old the battery is. This is all complicated stuff, and it actually isn't that important. You don't need to calculate the exact amounts of storage you need. What you need to do is get a rough estimate of what you need and then add on a little bit extra just to be safe.

Energy can also be stored in water. Water is very conductive of energy. This isn't energy you can convert into electricity, but by heating water, you are effectively storing thermal energy. When the sun is shining and you are pulling in a lot of power from your solar arrays, this is a great time to channel some of that energy into your water heater. Tanks with hot water will stay hot for a while. As we discussed, you're going to be pulling more energy in than you need at that time and more than you can store for later. Heating your water during the day is the perfect opportunity to store energy in the water.

Chapter 5:
Off-Grid Nutrition

Eating seems to be one of the most popular topics. That's for good reason: People love food. Plus, when you grow your own food, you have a more personal relationship with it. It's one thing to go to the store and pick up a zucchini; it's another thing entirely to grow that zucchini yourself from start to finish, see the final product, and then prepare it and feed it to yourself and other people.

A lot of people are very concerned about their food. Large agriculture corporations have earned themselves a bad reputation due to their practices of using pesticides and genetically modifying their crops in ways that are trade secrets. It's no surprise then that organic markets and farmers' markets have become so popular. What you eat is very important, and if you are especially alert about these things, there is no better way to know what you are eating than to be the person who makes it.

Growing Food

Gardening

You're certainly going to want a garden. If you aren't using a full-scale farming operation, a garden is a fantastic option. To maximize the value and productivity of that garden, we strongly recommended that you build a greenhouse. Greenhouses are less difficult to make than you might expect and have a few very important effects.

A garden inside of a greenhouse is less vulnerable to animals. If built correctly and securely, you won't have to worry about foxes and rabbits sneaking in and eating your greens.

Plants prefer warmer environments. The greenhouse contains both heat and moisture so that the plants are warm without drying out. The roof and walls protect the plants from the elements. Some plants are very sensitive to heavy rainfall, and several days of bad rain could wreck a garden. Depending on what you are growing ultimately depends on what the optimal temperature is. If you are going to be growing several plants at once, make sure that their optimal temperature overlaps so that all of them can be happy.

You want to keep the greenhouse relatively humid, but try not to break the 90% mark. Too much humidity could lead to mold. Likewise, at night, if things get too cold, humidity can turn to frost and freeze your plants, so make sure that you are maintaining the heat during the night as well.

Every garden should have a few staple items. For a beginner, it's best to stick with plants that aren't too needy. Since you can maximize the heat and water levels, the greenhouse will extend the natural planting season, and you will be able to get more food in one year than you would otherwise.

Vegetables that aren't a terrible amount of work include:

- any kind of hardy root vegetable, including carrots
- basil
- oregano
- tomatoes
- onions
- garlic
- cucumber
- zucchini
- lettuce
- spinach
- bell peppers
- celery

The French chefs reading this book probably noticed that all of the ingredients for mirepoix are present. Many Cajun chefs also noted that the Louisiana variation, "holy trinity," is also included on the list. Needless to say, you know you are off to a good start.

A garden that you plan on living off is a garden that produces all the things that you need to live—that means proteins, fats, antioxidants, and carbohydrates. Skipping out on any of these is not healthy.

If you're making a garden to survive then the nutritional values can be the most important thing. Your staples will include:

- potatoes
- carrots
- beans
- squash
- tomatoes
- onions
- corn

You want to mix and match your garden with foods that take little time to grow and also those that grow quickly. Then you can overlap the cycles of these two and have a constant set of nourishing plants being produced.

Some of the plants that have a short harvest cycle include:

- carrots
- kale
- spinach
- beans

All these will grow to full size within one to two months generally. Potatoes can take three to four months if you are using a spud from some of your older potatoes.

Vegetables don't last long. As soon as you pick them, their clock starts ticking. If you plan on doing a full harvest so that you can replant all of them, make sure you have a plan to consume them or at least a plan to store them. Effectively storing them will be covered later in this chapter.

If you can, you should also get a few herbs growing. A little bit of herb goes a long way, and you can grow most of them very easily. Basil, rosemary, sage, parsley, and thyme are all relatively simple and are excellent in food when they are fresh if you haven't tried it before.

The first part of running a garden is learning how to do it and getting it set up. The nice thing about plants is that most of the growing they do doesn't require much help from you. As long as you put them in a good environment with good soil, water, light, and the right temperature, they do all of the rest of the work.

If you want to get really fancy, you can integrate a greenhouse automation system. This requires a little bit of tactical know-how, but it will save you quite a bit of work in the long run.

By running pipes over your garden with small holes on it, with a time valve, you can have the garden automatically water itself. After the programmed period, water will automatically pump through the pipes and sprinkle the water out of the tiny holes, provided that you put the pipes in the right places. This automatic valve mechanism can be controlled via computer.

Another way to use computers is by ventilating your greenhouse. The temperature inside the greenhouse can't get too hot. Plants like hot temperatures but they have their limits. Using a computer to check the temperature and automatically turn on a fan to start ventilating the greenhouse is a great way of letting a machine do the micromanagement for you.

If you have a greenhouse, that's excellent, but if your garden is going to be too large to use in a greenhouse or you don't want a greenhouse for whatever reason, you are going to need to protect your garden from critters that will want to go in there and enjoy your snacks. Putting any kind of fencing around it so that rabbits and deer don't just wander in and enjoy themselves at your expense is necessary.

Raising Animals

Chickens

Chickens are great. Chickens will produce an egg every other day or so. The daily recommended minimum for protein consumption is about 50 grams. An egg contains about six grams of protein. So a breakfast of three eggs will contain about one-third of your daily required protein intake.

For chickens, you will absolutely need to build them a chicken coop. This usually entails an area fenced in with chicken wire with an indoor little home for them to sit comfortably. You can also let them out during the day— they know where their home is and will return. They'll love to look for bugs in your lawn, but you don't want them out all the time because they are very tasty treats for predators in the wild.

There is an increasing interest in raising home chickens or even ducks. You can find lengthy tutorials on how to raise these animals online. Even in places like Detroit, a lot of people have taken up urban farming projects and created chicken coops in the middle of the suburbs. Now is a great time to get into chicken farming on a small scale. There is so much support and information out there.

Chickens are very stupid and like to use their water as a bathroom. Change the water to make sure they don't kill themselves like that.

Chickens are great for laying eggs, but let us never forget that chickens are also great to eat. If you are raising organic, free-range chickens, you will be getting a very different product than what you might be used to at a grocery store. The ones you purchase at the store have been given growth hormones to make them huge, they get very little exercise, and they only "eat" rain. Your chickens will be considerably smaller but also way tastier. If you don't mind reducing your chicken consumption, you will have some extra tasty chicken as a reward.

A strange fact is that your chickens will seem to spontaneously die sometimes. You won't know why, and you can't afford a chicken autopsy. Don't be surprised when you come to your chicken village and find one of them didn't survive. That's just going to happen.

In any chicken coop, you will want one rooster. You do not want zero roosters, and you do not want two roosters. One rooster is exactly the right amount.

One rooster will be a good defender of the hens. If anyone tries to mess with their hands, the rooster will step in. If there are zero roosters, the hens are out of luck.

If you put two roosters next to each other, they will fight. This isn't a guess—that's what roosters do. The underground animal fighting sport known as cockfighting will happen literally every time you put two roosters next to each other. Roosters love to fight, and they will peck each other to death. Putting two roosters together may as well net you zero roosters.

Fish

If you have a pond or you want to build a pond, you can stock your own fish inside of it. These should be purchased from a decent fishery. You want to make sure that your fish are disease-free so that they won't get each other sick and die. Also, depending on the breed of fish that you were going with, you need to get the male to female ratio right. Otherwise, you might find it overpopulating too quickly, or you might find males fighting with one another depending on the species.

Your fish can be contained within a cage inside of the pond and makes it very easy to scoop them out with a net—not exactly like shooting fish in a barrel but very close.

Pigs

Pigs grow fast and will eat almost anything. They consume a lot of food, around six pounds a day, and will excrete one and a half pounds of waste. Since they'll eat almost anything, they will happily eat all of your leftover foods that are in table scraps, so they never have to go to waste.

Each pig is going to need at least 50 square feet of space and a pen that you build for them. You must keep the food and water far away from each other, optimally at opposite ends of the pen. They have a tendency to defecate near the water. If they start contaminating their own water supply, you're going to have to change it out. It's not good for them to be eating their own waste.

Pigs are very sensitive to sunlight. You can tell because they have very little fur and very light skin. You will definitely want to give them some kind of covering. Pigs usually protect their skin by rolling around the mud, but if they don't have mud because it is a particularly dry time or dry place, then they're going to need something else.

Once a pig has stopped gaining weight, usually at around 280 pounds or more, they are ready to eat. If you know how to butcher a pig or are willing to learn, that's great. Otherwise, you ought to contact a butcher who's close to you who can do that job for you safely and properly.

Pigs are very smart and very friendly. Not the wild ones: They will fight you. However, domesticated pigs are very friendly. There's been a growing trend where people even adopt pigs as family pets, just like dogs, and if you have not spent time around pigs, you may be surprised.

People who did not grow up on farms when they first encountered farm animals have a very different experience. People who grew up around animals and are accustomed to killing them and eating them have a very deep understanding of what meat is and where it comes from. They don't have any illusions about it. When most urban and suburban people see a chicken nugget, they don't think about it as it is.

When you spend time with a pig that you mean to ultimately slaughter and eat, it is understandable if you become emotionally attached. Your experience with animals has been probable that they are either pets or vermin. When the time comes, you might not feel good about killing the animal. There's no special advice on this, we're just warning you that this is a possibility. You can power through the experience and really confront what meat is, or you can decide you can't do it.

Goats

Goats are wonderful for milk, and they don't take up nearly as much room as cows. Some people really dislike goat milk while others think it's really great and are willing to pay a premium for it which is why you may see goat milk and cheese at a higher price at the store. Goats are sensitive to wind, and they need access to shade because they tend to overheat. Be sure to keep your goats and environment where they can keep cool.

Goats are natural lawn mowers. They will graze all day and keep your lawn trim. They can eat several pounds of food for a day just from grass and any hay that you supplement your diet with. They can also drink several gallons of water more or less depending on how much grazing they do, since a lot of their water needs are satisfied by grass.

If you are going to build them a place to live, that's a fantastic idea. They will want a place to sleep and be safe from predators and a place to keep the sun off of them— these shelters should probably be 70 square feet minimum.

There are a lot of things in nature that will poison your goat which they don't know better not to eat. Things like a poppy, stagger grass, and buckwheat are dangerous to a goat, so keep an eye on those.

Goats are also notorious climbers. Even domesticated goats love to climb things. A goat will even climb on top of other animals. Use an image search engine and look for yourself. Keep this in mind because if you have any way for the goat to get onto your roof, they might try to do that. If you are running solar panels on the roof, you probably don't want a goat walking around on them.

Rabbits

Rabbits are a classic option. You cannot survive on rabbit meat alone, however. There's a concept called rapid starvation which is also known as protein poisoning and is caused by the overconsumption of protein with no fat carbohydrates or micronutrients. Rabbits are perfectly fine as are any other lean game so long as you are keeping them part of a well-balanced diet.

Rabbits don't require a lot of space, which is nice. They are extremely good at escaping, though. Your rabbit cage needs to be tighter than Alcatraz, otherwise they will get out. Rabbits are natural diggers, so you'll need to make sure that you have some caging on the ground or floor, so they don't get out that particular way.

Also, rabbits are cute. If you are going to get cold feet and not want to butcher them, that's fine—you can always keep them as pets. However, don't let the rabbit breeding get out of control, which is something that can easily happen if you aren't careful. Breeding is great if you're making food for stew but it's not good when suddenly you have way more pets than you know what to do with. The same situation goes with pigs.

Turkey

Turkeys are an all-American bird, and you can purchase them from a turkey breeder or farm for very cheap. Turkeys are very sensitive animals, and you are likely to lose several of the first few weeks after you buy them. Chicks need to have a warming unit when they are, such as 100–250W lamps. They need to keep the battery at about 100 degrees Fahrenheit for the first week—they want to be toasty. After the first week, they are much less vulnerable, and you can gradually reduce the heat; after a few months, they won't need any heat at all.

Turkeys grow fast, and after three and a half months, they will be big enough that they are ready to be eaten. At 35–45 pounds, they are a lot of food, so be sure to have a way to store the meat properly, or share it with others. There's a reason why a turkey is a traditional bird for Thanksgiving—many people sitting together are all able to share a meal together.

Turkeys are also very smelly. You do not want turkeys anywhere near your house or upwind of it. They also aren't terribly friendly. Unlike some of the other animals, they are not good pets, but they are good food.

Unlike pigs and chickens, there is no way you will get emotionally attached to a turkey. To be perfectly frank, they are mean and their odor is very pungent. If you are maybe squeamish about killing an animal, maybe a turkey is a good way to start because you will not feel bad at all.

Bees

If you have a sweet tooth, you could even consider raising bees. This is an insect that is absolutely vital to the ecosystem and great if you like sugar. Honey is the only known food that never goes bad. There is nothing that you need to do with a container of honey to maintain it. Honey never rots. Honey will retain its edibility longer than you will be alive.

Beekeeping is a very popular hobby. It also has two wonderful side effects: It will produce honey and will pollinate your garden. The easiest way to get started with a beekeeping operation is to purchase the basic starter kits. These are not difficult to find on the Internet. A starter kit usually contains everything you need: frames, a hive feeder, a queen excluder, a smoker, and all your protective gear.

You can keep your bees within a quarter-mile of your garden, and they will do all the work of pollinating your plants. Also depending on where you place them can affect the flavor of the honey. Putting bees next to cloves will add a clove flavor to the honey.

It's a fun hobby and does require some research because there's a lot more to it than you might think. Honey can also be a cool gift. If you put it in a jar and give it to someone, it's a neat and personal thing.

Another by-product of raising bees is wax which can be used for sealing, protecting food to extend life, and making candles.

Dogs

No, we're not suggesting that you eat dog meat! They are just included here because we're already discussing animals. You're not going to eat the bees either.

Dog people are lucky. An off-grid lifestyle is wonderful for dogs. They have tons of space to move around, and they don't need to be taken on walks because there's nowhere for them to run off to.

Dogs also love just to spend time with people while they're working outside, which you will be doing plenty of. Dogs are essentially wolves that were genetically engineered through selective breeding to become home security systems. In a city, you'll find dogs bark at almost any noise that they hear. They bark at people walking by on the sidewalk or another dog a block away that is heading toward the sidewalk. Deep in the country, that response is important. If you are isolated, it's unlikely that you will have unwelcome human visitors, but you can certainly expect unwelcome animal visitors. This could be foxes coming to eat your chickens. This could be a bear simply wandering through. It could be a raccoon who has sniffed out your trash. Whatever it may be, dogs have extremely sharp senses of smell in hearing and will know if you have welcomed visitors long before you do, and they will eagerly tell you about it.

Foods to Grow/Stock up On

Food storage is immensely important. Humans have developed many clever ways of keeping their food clean and safe long before refrigeration.

There are a few foods that are always good to have on hand. Even if you aren't living off-grid, it is just smart to have these in your home.

Rice

Rice has a long shelf life, and if properly stored, rice can last six months or longer. If you also keep it refrigerated, you can get twice as much time out of it. Brown rice is a great source of vitamins and fiber. Brown rice is the most nutritious, and if you're eating to stay alive, just go where the nutrition is.

Price is a staple food for more than half of the planet. That's a pretty ringing endorsement.

Beans

The best friend to rice is beans. This is a well-known and well-traveled survival food. It's also very versatile and can be used in a lot of different ways. Dried beans can be stored for a long time and can be hydrated rather quickly just by soaking and heating them.

Beans are an excellent source of protein, and when complemented with rice, it forms a complete protein.

Nuts

They are an excellent source of protein and fat; dried nuts also store very well.

Cabbage

Yes, cabbage. It is low in calories, but it has a ton of nutrients including B6 and C, and it is very fibrous. It's also very versatile because it can be used in salads. If you are into pickling, you can turn it into sauerkraut or kimchi, which is a great flavor addition and has a very good shelf life.

Corn

It's very easy to grow as long as the soil temperature stays high enough to allow for germination, and you have mature soil. If you can get those two things right, corn is very easy to grow.

Cucumbers

If you plan on pickling, you should have cucumbers. If you are just getting cucumbers for pickling, keep in mind that there is a specific type of cucumber called a pickling cucumber. The ordinary cucumber you're used to that you put on a salad does not work the same way, but you might also like regular cucumbers.

Potatoes

Everybody loves potatoes. It's a starchy crop that's high in carbohydrates, which is important for getting your calorie intake high enough. These are crops that you are trying to live off of, and calories are your body's fuel. Yukon Gold potatoes are probably the best choice.

Sweet Potatoes

Everything we just said about potatoes is true of sweet potatoes. They are calorie dense and have much more iron nutrient content than your average potato. The leafy greens that grow on them are also edible. They have a longer growing season, longer than almost anything else you will be raising. However, if you like sweet potatoes, they might be worth the extra time and effort.

Tomatoes

Setting aside the argument about whether it is a fruit or a vegetable, the tomato is a pretty easy plant as long as you give it ample water. They also like the temperature on the warm side. Tomatoes are great on so many things and can be turned into sauces, added to salads, added on top of burgers, and plenty of other applications.

Lentils

Lentils are packed with protein. It's very difficult to get a decent amount of protein from plant sources: Ask any vegetarian who is conscious of their nutrition. Lentils have around 18 grams of protein per serving—that is the same amount of protein as three eggs. Also, lentils are one of the oldest crops that have ever been cultivated by humans. It is ancient, and lentil soup is just delicious, so if you don't like lentils, start liking lentils.

Spinach

This plant is very easy to grow and packed with vitamins and minerals. For the adventurous, spinach can be stored by freezing it or dehydrating it and then crushing it into a powder. Now you have a powdered nutritional supplement available.

Berries

Everybody loves berries. Raspberries, cranberries, blueberries, or whatever kind of berry. They're all good. They have a lot of nutrition, they have a natural sweetness, and you can do a lot with them. You can turn them into jelly and incorporate them into nearly any dessert item you can think of.

Dry Seasoning and Salt

There's no reason to not make your food taste good even in an emergency or disaster situation. Always have seasoning. There's no good reason not to. Dried herbs and spices last a really long time.

Dehydrating, Salting, and Smoking

For food to go bad, it needs to be wet. Salting food increases the acidity and also dries it out, which in tandem makes bacteria grow much slower. This is exactly why beef jerky was invented. Salted meats have been with humans for as long as we've had salt.

For those who really enjoy food and want to go the extra mile, you should consider building a smokehouse. The process of smoking food adds a wonderful flavor that's impossible to replicate and also dries out the food which helps to preserve it. Smoked salmon, for example, is delicious and a fantastic source of protein.

You can dehydrate meats, but you can also dehydrate fruits. It's also a good idea to put a type of acid on it such as lemon juice or another citrus because the drawing process takes a while. You want to prevent any bacteria from starting a home there during the process.

There are plenty of ways to dry food, including the inside of an oven, or you could have a special dehydrator that uses electricity. One good option is to use a nonelectric dehydrator. It's hard to measure exactly how much time you need to dehydrate any kind of food because depending on your environment, it will change a lot. The outside temperature, humidity, and amount of wind passing through will greatly alter these times. It should take six hours minimum but can take a lot more depending on the thickness and what it is you are dehydrating in the environment. With that being said, you should check in on your dehydration regularly.

Dehydrating doesn't need to use any electricity. Solar dehydrators are a great method, which uses the sun itself to dehydrate. As long as you have a rack to place the food on, make sure that they are ventilated, they are stacked accordingly, and have netting around to keep any bugs off of it, it's not too difficult.

There are many different designs to this sort of thing— one is to create a flat box with a mesh to lay food on then cover it with a metal covering. The sun will heat up the metal, raising the internal temperature. As long as there's proper ventilation underneath it to allow moisture to escape, this is a very simple DIY method.

You can dehydrate beef and fish but DO NOT try to dehydrate birds or pigs. Exposing those kinds of animals to air for longer than is absolutely necessary is extremely dangerous. Do not do it.

Pickling and Canning

There's been a recent new interest in recreational pickling and canning. These are excellent ways to preserve her food. Pickling also has the advantage of adding a vinegar flavor to whatever you want.

You can do just about anything, including meat. Things that are canned need to be sealed properly, so double-check it. Once canned, they need to be stored properly in a cool place without too much sunlight. This could mean a pantry or shed. If you are in a warmer temperature climate, you should seriously consider digging a cellar. The heat of the sun doesn't penetrate very far into the earth, and if you dig down just a short way, you can make a permanently cool space.

If a cellar is too much, it is totally fine if you want to bury your food. A hole in the ground, covered up, will be a natural refrigerator and keep the sun off and hopefully away from animals.

Cooling

Some kinds of foods absolutely need to be stored in a cool place. Some can be left at room temperature, you probably know which ones those are already. According to the FDA, certain foods will require refrigeration and that temperature needs to be 40 degrees Fahrenheit or less. That's very close to freezing temperature. During the winter, you don't need to worry about this that much because if it is already 40 degrees and cold around, then nature is doing your refrigeration for you.

In the summer, you are going to need to find other ways of storing your meat, poultry, fish, dairy, certain cooked foods, eggs, and all the rest.

Certain foods you already know you can leave out are your coffee, bread, onions, honey, olive oil, and potatoes—these are all fine.

The oldest traditional method is to simply build a root cellar. A hole in the ground will be much cooler than the surface or the inside of your home during the summer.

If necessary, you can always go with the old-fashioned route of getting a cooler. If you don't plan on ever storing your food for particularly long, some of the newer and more expensive coolers are extremely good at retaining cold temperature.

If you make a mistake and don't do a good job of preserving your food, look for the following symptoms: nausea, diarrhea, abdominal pain, fever, and vomiting. If you are suffering from one or more of those symptoms, especially if other people in your home are after eating the same thing, you need to reach out and contact medical help immediately—you may be suffering from food poisoning. This can be very dangerous, as it's more than just a stomachache.

Whatever food preservation method or methods you use, don't take any chances with your own health. If food looks iffy, don't take risks.

A really nice, well-insulated chest freezer and/or refrigerator are great. They use less electricity than you might expect, just as long as you don't have kids who like to hang out with the door open, looking at every single thing in the fridge. Don't get a cheap fridge or freezer. A really great, well-insulated fridge pays for itself.

How to Feed Yourself Without Power

Electric ovens crave using as much energy as possible. You cannot use an electric stove, as it is simply not realistic. Likewise, microwaves can be very power-hungry, too. They might be fine to use when you are running at peak energy intake, and you have sunshine and wind, but it's not a great method. Electric stoves are terrible anyway, so nothing is lost. There are plenty more electrically conservative ways to cook that are simply better for cooking.

Wood Stove

If you already have a wood stove in your house keeping you warm, why not cook on it, too? This is a very old and rustic way of cooking food, but it served our ancestors well for hundreds of years. The same fire that's heating up your home also has a flat surface on top. You can simply put a pot on it or a skillet, and do your best to control the temperature by controlling the fire. It's not using any more power than it was before, so there's no reason not to utilize this.

Now it's the middle of summer, so you probably don't want to be having a piping hot fire in your living room. Try to avoid that heat as much as possible; during the summer, you are going to want to stay far away from any kind of fire, and try one of the other options.

Solar Oven

A solar oven is a kind of box with mirrors on the inside and a couple of sides missing. Basically, it's a big shiny device that catches solar energy and then points it into a focal point inside of it. Whatever you want to cook, you simply place it inside the container in that focal point. On a sunny day, this will heat up whatever you are cooking very quickly. Think about when you touch metal on a hot day and how hot that gets.

This type of cooking is probably not great for everything. It is excellent for anything that you need to cook slowly or something that doesn't need to be cooked at a high temperature. For example, you are not going to be cooking steaks or kebabs on one of these things. Instead, any kind of stew would be excellent, or any kind of vegetable that you can cook slowly would be a great way to go. This is a completely green, powerless slow cooker.

There's no way to turn the temperature up or down or to regulate in any particular way, so your best option is to check on a frequency or to place it in such a spot that after enough time, the shadow will cover it and essentially turn it off.

Propane

For cooking, you can use tanks of gas. This is just like a propane tank on a grill that you would use outside. The only difference is that it is a built-in device in your home and also contains an oven. You can't cultivate propane on your own land, which means you will need to purchase it elsewhere or have it delivered.

Gas is great for cooking and is the preferred heating element for the best chefs. It's also relatively cheap if you are just using it for cooking and not trying to heat your entire home with it.

Grilling

Just as simple as that: Everybody knows how to grill, and everybody loves grilling.

If you're using propane to grill, that's going to require you to have propane on hand. If you already happen to have propane running in your kitchen, that is very handy. If you are a charcoal kind of person, that is a great option. Charcoal doesn't go bad. You can store that for as long as you like.

Grilling means great flavor and the outdoor tradition. With a large enough surface, you can prepare a lot of food at the same time. That makes it always a great option if you have a lot of guests or a large family.

If you are raising pigs or you are doing any hunting, a pellet grill is a fantastic option for cooking large amounts of meat. Slowly add in little pellets of wood pulp—they look a lot like hamster food. This keeps feeding a fire at exactly the right amounts to maintain a steady temperature. You can get a slow cooking process going, then you wait 12 hours, culminating in an unbelievably tasty and tender meal the next day, with very little effort.

Earth Oven

Earth ovens are excellent options. You need a slab of stone, and you're going to house that using rocks and dirt to create something like a mound with a mouth on one side that food could be inserted into. Beneath, you can put in some lumber to burn. These things, once they're cooking, get ridiculously hot. The work on it is a very efficient way to insulate the heat, and very little gets wasted even with the open side. If you pop an oven into this, it will be fully cooked in just a few minutes.

During the summer months when you want to keep your home as cool as possible, cooking outside is a great way to make sure that the heat stays outside. From a cooking and aesthetic frame, earth ovens are just cool. You can cook food crazy fast.

They lend themselves to cooking certain kinds of food very well which, if you are into cooking, is a fun culinary experiment. Also, they happen to be very easy to build. Anyone can make one with a few simple instructions. They're all so very cheap because mostly what you need is brick and dirt.

Living off the Land

Depending on your environment and your personal ethics, you can do what people have done for millennia. Nature readily provides protein in the form of animals. Hunting is certainly an option that you can avail yourself of if you want.

This isn't a book about hunting, and we won't go into deep detail about it, but if it is something you're interested in, there are plenty of resources available so that you can learn more about the topic.

States and counties have many laws regarding hunting, fishing, and trapping, and you will need to learn them to not break any laws.

Don't Eat Wild Mushrooms

This should go without saying but some people don't know: Do NOT eat wild mushrooms. We cannot say this strongly enough. We don't care if you have a book on identifying mushrooms. Unless you are a mycologist, do not go putting wild mushrooms in your mouth. Mushrooms can be very dangerous. Even with photographs, the differences between a safe one and a dangerous one can be indistinguishable.

Also, don't eat berries. Don't eat things in the woods if you don't know what you're doing.

Hunting

Hunting with a gun usually has a very short season. There are considerations about what kinds of animals you can hunt during which portion of the season. An average size buck can net you an average of 60 or 70 pounds of meat. A boar can net you double that, which is a lot of meat. You should have some friends or a good way to store it.

If you're using more difficult means of hunting, such as a bow or a black powder rifle, you will have a larger season to hunt in.

If you live in a remote area that has dangerous wildlife such as bears or cougars, having a form of self-defense might be very valuable. Bear spray and other nonlethal weapons are good to have, but if your concern is protecting yourself from a mama bear who feels threatened by you, you're going to want the best tool that you can avail yourself of. This can mean a 10mm pistol at your side or a strong hunting rifle chambered in something like 6.5mm Creedmoor.

Most animals are not interested in you and will not pick a fight with you. However, starving and desperate animals might take their chances; an animal that perceives you as a threat to their young might attack you. These kinds of attacks don't happen often, but when they do, they are brutal. People are torn apart and isolated in the wilderness and unable to easily contact medical aid.

A well-placed shot will kill an animal so quickly that they are dead before they realize what has happened. Taking a bad shot and wounding an animal is a serious faux pas among hunters. Hunters do not want to hurt animals: They want to hunt animals. Wounding an animal is cruel, and tracking a wounded animal to finish the job is not anyone's idea of fun.

If you are interested in hunting but are not experienced, your best bet is to make friends with someone who is. There are a lot of things to learn, not just the laws, of which any good hunter will be well aware. There's also considerations like how to safely harvest what you need, how to most humanely kill an animal, how to stay downwind of an animal, or how to transport the animal after it has been shot. There are many things you should familiarize yourself with before you go walking around in the woods with a gun and no idea what you are doing.

Fishing

Fishing is a great form of recreation and the catch you get will be a great form of protein. If you have access to water that has edible fish, that can be a great asset. Depending on where you live, you might have fishing options all over. You aren't locked to your property, remember. There may be great lakes and streams close enough that you can walk or drive and get yourself a meal—with a fishing license, naturally.

For the truly committed fish eater, you can build an artificial pond and populate it with your own supply of fish. With a river, you can trap fish with zero effort and come by and pick them up as you like.

Trapping

Trapping is a tricky business but has been a staple for eons. Trapping doesn't mean those terrifying spiky metal claws, like bear traps. Those are illegal, so do not use them. If you have one, we don't know where you found one, but don't use it.

Trapping usually means cages and snares. Once again, this is something that depends on your local law, and you need to investigate it before you get involved. The advantage of trapping is that you don't need to do anything other than set up the traps and visit them occasionally. This generates a passive supply of animals without the work of chasing.

It's simply pieces of twine that are attached in certain strategic locations.

If you are tracking, you may be able to find common routes for rabbits. If they find a path that they like, they will keep using it, knowing that it is a relatively safe trail. However, if you know about it, too, it is not so safe for them. A live trap or a snare in one of these spots could nab you a bunny.

If you are the kind of person that isn't squeamish about eating squirrels, just know that they are very easy to catch in a snare. Simply by taking a piece of wood and leaning against a tree, squirrels are lazy like all animals and take the path of least resistance. Squirrels always walk up the branch leaning against the tree which makes a branch the perfect place to leave a snare.

Whatever traps you have on your property, you should be checking them a couple times a day just to make sure to see if anything is there. Snaring and trapping is a game of numbers. The more traps you have set out, the more likely you are to catch any animal.

Snare traps are cheap, but live traps are easy. Just simply get a cage that will close itself when something goes inside of it. Bait that with something the animal of your preference likes and visit to see if anyone took the bait.

Chapter 6:
Heating and Cooling Your off-Grid Home

Heating and cooling are easy to leave as afterthoughts until the moment you need them. If the temperature gets too hot or too cold, you will be miserable. If it gets bad enough, it can be lethal. There are a lot of options here, which is nice.

To be perfectly honest, if a lot of things aren't going great, you can put up with it. If you have to haul your water out or if you can't get your garden running so you have to continue to go to the grocery store, those are all things that you can live with. However, if you are living in a home that is 95 degrees Fahrenheit for a solid week straight, you are going to abandon this project as soon as you can. No one can be expected to live like that when there is a cozy Holiday Inn just 25 miles away.

If your temperature is off, everything else will be off, too, so this is one thing you definitely need to get right.

If you have animals, don't forget them! If you are hot, they are hot; if you are cold, they are cold.

Heating and Cooling

What's better than having a heating system and a cooling system? Having a system that both helps heating and cooling at the same time. Geothermal and passive solar designs are great for all kinds of temperature regulation, both hot and cold. They should be integrated into the home when it's built. Retrofitting a house after the fact might cost you more money and trouble than it's worth. These are integral to the house and are both fantastic systems.

Geothermal

We already discussed geothermal concerning energy in a previous chapter, so we don't want to repeat too much of what was there. Geothermal is outstanding for temperature control because it draws on air that is always cooler than the air when it is hot outside and is always warmer than the air when it is freezing outside.

Geothermal works by running a winding series of pipes underground, then, they draw water through those pipes with a pump that will enter into your home. Sometimes, these pipes will run through the floor and the walls.

The upfront costs can be high, but it is one of the most energy-efficient options for keeping the temperature out of your home comfortably.

After you dig 10 feet under the ground. It's always 55 degrees Fahrenheit, no matter what time of year it is. If it's 100 degrees out, 10 feet down is 55 degrees. It gets to be -10 outside, 10 feet down, it's still 55 degrees.

Geothermal heating system runs water at this temperature and is then able to transmit it to the air using water pumps and fans. This uses some electricity but much less than a standard heating or cooling system.

Depending on the space this can cost several thousands to build, so it will also save a lot of money if you put it together yourself. This isn't too difficult but does require a lot of work.

Geothermal is a very cool system, and there isn't any home that wouldn't benefit from a geothermal system.

Passive Solar Design

Passive solar design is clever architecture and a design of building itself to maximize heat when you need it and minimize heat when you want it to be cooler.

There's a very important mosque in Israel called the Dome of the Rock. It is considered very important and has a very clever design. The mosque is a large stone dome. When the sun rises, it begins to heat up the rock, but it takes a while for this heat to penetrate the stone and reach the inside. By the time it is beginning to heat up the mosque, enough time has passed that the sun is already beginning its descent on the Western horizon. Then, throughout the night, the stone that was used up all day cools, and by the morning, the schedule repeats itself. By simply having a dome of exactly the right amount of stone, it can keep the occupants of the mosque comfortable even in the tremendous scorching summers of the Middle East.

Passing solar design in a modern house uses techniques like this. By choosing exactly where the windows are, facing them toward the sunlight at particular times of day can make an enormous impact. Choosing where to place awnings so that the sunlight will not get in through windows, depending on where it is in the sky, also has a major impact. The particular place you choose to keep a wood-burning stove or trees around the property in the home and how that blocks out sunlight is also a huge factor.

Any kind of passive solar design will be completely integrated with the house. It has to take into account that the direction to the Sun is the height of the Sun during the summer and during the winter. We need to factor in things like the direction that the wind blows. It needs to take into consideration the trees and hills nearby. A good passive solar design will be completely customized for that particular environment, so two houses with passive solar designs will often look very different depending on where they are.

For that reason, passive solar design is a little bit like feng shui. You probably aren't going to know how to do it, and if it's something that interests you, you are going to need to learn a heck of a lot of things before you attempt it yourself. Alternatively, you can reach out and look for architects or contractors who are familiar with passive solar design, and you can help you come up with something that you are happy with.

For the sake of this book, we can't go into too much depth about solar design because that could be an entire book in itself. However, you are encouraged to look into it if you are designing your own home. You can get a lot of interesting ideas that cost you next to nothing but will make your heating and cooling considerably cheaper.

Heating Your Home

Wood Stove

Probably the most popular way to eat your home would be with the classic stove fireplace. These are just lovely to look at, and seeing fire gives off a cozy atmosphere. Many of these can also be used as a stovetop where pots can be placed directly on top to cook with. These things get extremely hot, so this might not be a good option if you have small children.

To operate these things, you also need to clean them regularly, and you will need to get firewood. Firewood can be found, purchased, made, and would need to be kept dry. Wood also needs to be prepared, so large logs should be split into halves, quarters, and thin smaller pieces.

You'll need a chimney, and if you have small children, you will absolutely need a barrier of some kind to keep your kids away. These things get HOT, and no one wants to see a toddler get a bad burn by touching one of these.

They come in all varieties, some very traditional and some very modern. Wood stoves give really warm energy, and we don't just mean heat. They have a certain vibe that they give to a room.

You'll need firewood way ahead of actually needing wood. That means, you need your wood chopped, dry, and in large supply well ahead of when you plan on burning it. Green, freshly cut wood doesn't burn well, and it kicks out sparks. Put your wood someplace dry. Building a barrier over a woodpile to keep the rain off is basically mandatory. Also, you should have your logs already chopped into quarters and smaller bits. The small pieces will be needed as kindling to get the fire going, and once it's cooking, you'll want to be feeding this fire with quarter logs or at least halves. if you are chilling on a cold, winter night, you don't want to have to make a trip outside to chop wood.

Two major drawbacks of the woodfire stove are that they need to be cleaned regularly. You're going to have to get in there with a shovel and remove all of the ash. It's inside your house, so you have to be careful not to get gray dust onto everything. Ashes are a good source of compost, so be sure to add them to anything you want to use to grow.

The other drawback of the woodfire stove is, of course, fire safety. If you aren't careful about managing the fire to a good level and it gets too big or if there's some kind of congestion in the chimney, you can find your house filling with smoke or starting a fire. No matter whether you have a woodfire stove or not, you should own a fire extinguisher. You are probably living far away from any fire department. Everyone needs a fire extinguisher, and that's doubly true if you are building fires inside your home.

Compost Water Heater

Compost heating sounds pretty gross, but if you do it right, don't worry: It won't be gross at all. As organic material breaks down, part of the process is that as microorganisms break down the material, their life cycle releases heat. Compost heating captures this heat and moves it into a conductive source such as water, and then, you can use that water as it is almost warm, or you can pump it through a system to heat up your home.

A compost pile of wood chips can actually put out a considerable amount of heat. You'll notice it because usually these things are left outdoors, and the heat dissipates immediately. A good compost heap gets hotter than you might think.

Running pipes through a compost heats the same way that you would for geothermal, achieving a similar effect. The heat is transferred into the pipe water. The heat is there, all you have to do is capture it. You can also use this water to heat a greenhouse if you are using one or through a radiant heat floor system. You can even find instances of people using it to heat up a hot tub all year. In the last chapter of this book, we'll go into greater detail about how to compost, but for now, it's sufficient to mention that a compost pile will get very hot, up to 150 degrees Fahrenheit. That is much hotter than most people would feel comfortable relaxing in.

Radiant Heat Floor

If you can heat up a lot of water using composting or solar energy, try radiant floor heating. Radiant floor heating looks a lot like compost heating and geothermal but in reverse. The way it works is that hot water is run in piping that zigzags underneath the floor. The pipes touch aluminum plating which is attached to wood. Simply having the pipes making contact with the metal and wood transmits the heat, and a small amount of heat generates upward from the floor. Since heat rises, it creates a general, warm, and ambient temperature. Also because it's just spread out, there are no fans necessary. The heat doesn't just turn on and off based on what a thermometer reads.

A system like this requires a lot of piping and specially made floors. They also need a reliable pump system to keep the water moving.

People spend good money to enjoy heated flooring systems in their bathrooms. These have become very popular with those that can afford them. The radiant floor heating works on the same principle but is much cooler than the bathroom heating. They just heat one room, but you can heat your whole house. Incidentally, if you have a pet cat, they will love this.

Cooling Your Home

It's easier to warm up than it is to cool off. Keeping cool is a very tricky business that has been with humans for the entire history of our species. Our ancestors had to find solutions with much fewer resources and technology than we have now.

One of the considerations for where you choose to live will certainly involve your heat tolerance. Some people feel comfortable in warm environments, and other people just sweat, melt, and feel miserable. Managing your heat is super important. You're going to be feeling pretty miserable if you move out to your new home and are deteriorating in 90-degree weather all summer long.

Thankfully, some options are relatively power efficient and won't require a lot of electricity.

Air Conditioning

One of the greatest modern inventions ever made is the air conditioner. We tend to think of it as a luxury good, but it has had a profound impact on human life.

Water is extremely conductive. That means electricity passes through it easily, and it collects heat easily. Imagine if you put a pot of water in the oven and set the temperature to 500 degrees Fahrenheit, letting it sit for a couple hours. If you were to reach your hand into the oven, you would feel the heat in your hand, but it wouldn't burn you immediately. If you put your hand in the bucket, you would cook your hand. The water is very conductive, but the air isn't.

The way your body manages heat is by sweating. Since water is conductive, and saltwater is extra conductive, the heat stays in the sweat as it leaves the body. The sweat falls off or dries away, carrying the heat with it. Air conditioning works the same way, in principle, using a compressor and an expansion valve filled with refrigerant fluid.

You've seen your electric bills in the summer, so you already know that air conditioners are very expensive to keep running—these are electrically hungry machines.

That said, if the sun is shining and heating you up, they are also feeding your solar systems if you have one. This means that air conditioners are a ripe instance where you can take advantage of opportunity usage, which we covered earlier in the chapter about generating power. If you have enough solar power feeding your air conditioner, the sheets that are making you boil are the exact same energy that is going to cool you down.

Solar Chimney

Solar chimneys work on a very clever principle. You run a black pipe through the roof just like any other chimney, tap it off so that rainfall won't come in it, and put a grate in it so that animals won't climb down it. Since the pipe is black, it will absorb more solar energy and heat it up. Likewise, the air inside of the pipe will also heat up. Hot air rises. When the air in the pipe begins to rise up, it creates a suction effect that pulls air up out of the house itself.

On another portion or portions of the house, there is also great air intake. There's always somewhere that is relatively cool—this could be in the shade or from your geothermal system. Since the hot air at the chimney is creating a suction effect and pulling air through the house, the new air will come in through the cold vents, or the geothermal system does add cool air into the home.

These systems are very different from your traditional methods. Some people have great success with these, and others don't. It's certainly something that requires thought and planning to maximize its benefits.

The major drawback of this design is that you cannot retrofit a building—it has to be designed as an integral part of the architecture.

Solar Fans

You can't go wrong with fans. Fans are cheap and don't require a lot of power. In fact, when you need to fan the most, the sun is usually shining. Solar fans are often a very good option. Fans inside of an animal's space will help keep them cool and also help ventilate any smells. It's also recommended that solar fans be placed inside any greenhouse that you build. This will help regulate the temperature inside. Plants like it hot, but they don't like it too hot.

If you're clever about it, you can find cool spaces near your house, using a fan to blow the cool air in and a different fan to push the hot air out. You can run a pipe or something through a shady area for your intake fan. You can also run an output fan at a higher level where the hottest air goes.

This is a very low-tech solution. We would not recommend using this alone. This is a good way to supplement any other cooling system that you have, but it probably won't be sufficient on its own, just like rainwater is insufficient to cover all of your water needs.

Sun Oven and Outdoor Fires

On a hot day, you do not want to be cooking food indoors. All the heat produced will just make your home that much hotter. Cooking outside is a great solution. It's no accident that summer is the grilling season.

Sun Oven is the perfect product to reduce the indoor heat. It's a box with a couple open sides and reflective surfaces on the inside. This works exactly as you would expect. The sun reflects and cooks whatever you place inside the Sun Oven. It's not fast—it works like a slow cooker, which makes it great for stews and chili.

Chapter 7:
Off-Grid Waste Management

Waste management is very important and also one of the things we think about least when considering living off the grid. When you live on a plumbing and sewage system and have garbage collection regularly, you don't have to think about this very much. However, when waste disposal becomes your job to take care of, you will understand how important it really is.

DO NOT dump your septic waste on your property. It is gross, illegal, and dangerous. We're sure most of my readers already know this, but for the rest of you, don't do this. We don't care if animals use the wilderness as their restroom.

Trash and Composting

Any leftover material that you are throwing out such as scraps from dinner, leftover food that goes bad, or little bits of meat on the bones of ribs you cooked the night before can be used to fuel your garden.

There's no need to waste perfectly good material. Even things like coffee grounds, eggshells, and ash can be great in a garden. You will definitely want to have a separate place to dispose of compostable materials and set that aside. If you own pigs, they are always happy to have any scraps or leftovers that you are done with.

If you're doing any gardening, and you probably are, you are going to definitely want a compost pile.

There are two kinds of composting: hot and cold. Cold is as simple as taking the waste and putting it in a container or pile and letting them decompose.

Hot composting requires more work, but it speeds up the process. When the weather is warm, you can speed it up so that it is done in a month or two. To get faster composting, you're going to need oxygen, water, carbon, and nitrogen. All of these things will help feed the microorganisms that will consume the matter, speeding up the rate of decay.

You can also speed this up by purchasing worms. You won't be using the night crawlers that you buy for fishing or any other worm. Specifically, you need red worms, also sometimes called red wigglers. These are not hard to find. Any place that has a decent gardening supply section should be able to help you out.

Whatever the bio trash you are using, you are also going to want to add nitrogen-rich material. This would include grass trimmings, leaves, tree branches, newspaper, hay, cardboard, and wood chips. Any of these materials should be mixed in with the material you are composting.

If you aren't getting much rain, you're going to need to water the pile regularly just like it's a garden of trash. You're not trying to get totally soaked—you just want to add enough water that the microorganisms can do their job. However, don't add so much that you drown your red wigglers. If you can put your hand inside of it and feel it's producing a lot of heat, you are doing it right.

About every week or so, you should turn your pile over and let it mix around. To do this with the shovel or pitchfork, just keep it moving. Make sure it's getting oxygen in the center. At this point, it should be getting very hot, up to 150 degrees.

Your compost is done when it stops putting out lots of heat. It should start looking like dirt again. At that point, it is perfect for your garden, so go ahead and transplant that dirt and all your red wigglers into their new home.

Trash

Anything that isn't compostable, biodegradable, or burnable, such as plastic, should be placed in a container and set aside. Since you don't have a trash removal service coming to your location, you will need to take it to a dump yourself or schedule someone to come and get it. Hopefully, the amount of this kind of waste will diminish over time, and these trips will become less frequent.

Burn

Some things are perfectly fine to burn such as wood or cotton, cloth, paper towel rolls, and dryer lint. Again, just like the water, don't set anything on fire that is going to create toxicity. Don't try burning plastic or metal with paint on it or something else that you wouldn't want to breathe.

When burning things, always do so responsibly. Don't start a fire if you live in a dry climate during a dry spell. In certain places like Wyoming and Colorado, starting fires can be very risky. If you are going to use a burn barrel, just be careful, and be sure to have a fire extinguisher close by.

We're sure we sound like a broken record but here it is: Make sure it is legal to burn your trash. Different places have different rules. If you're deep enough back from the road, probably no one will see you, but it needs to be said.

Gray Water

Gray water is dirty water from your sink or shower—this isn't toilet water. It's simple enough to get rid of so long as you aren't using soaps and detergents with harmful chemicals. If you are using all-natural stuff to wash your body and your dishes, then this water can simply be grounded out of the house and dropped onto the soil working to be reabsorbed by the earth. Be sure that nothing you deposit is going to be harmful and harm the plants or wildlife out there or be something that you don't want anything to do with the groundwater.

Make sure nothing that goes into the gray water is harmful. You can check all your labels and investigate if you have any doubts. If you are using detergents and soaps that are harmful, you can always put those into a septic system.

Depending on how you set up your water, there are many ways to capture your gray water and separate it from your septic system. It can be simply diverted into a bucket. As simple as that sounds, that's completely viable. Gray water could also be diverted toward a particular use that you have in mind. For example, gray water, provided that it is clean enough that it won't hurt plants, could potentially be diverted into the yard to be reabsorbed by the soil. If you are especially confident of the quality of your gray water, you could even divert it to your garden to water plants.

Gray water that is dirty can also be used for flushing toilets, washing your clothes, or washing your car. That is a good way to get multiple uses out of one batch of water and get much more efficient use for it. That's definitely more preferable than dumping it in a septic system.

Septic System

Probably the most popular option is to install a septic system. If you have any kind of internal plumbing in your home, you are definitely going to need this. A septic system is a gigantic tank buried underground just like a water tank, but instead of holding water, it holds everything you flush down the toilet. We don't want the septic system boiling, and we don't want it freezing. Either is going to be a worse disaster than bursting the water tanks, believe me.

Tanks have a hatch, and you will need to periodically have a waste removal truck come and suck out of the waste that is stored there. Depending on the size of your tank and how many people live in your home, this could be only once every few years.

Outhouse

Outhouses are a very old way of doing things. They don't require any water and are very easy to build. It may not be surprising to know that most people don't want to use an outhouse. To use the bathroom you're going to have to leave your house, and if it's in the dead of winter, that's not too fun.

If you don't want to live a life within our house, they might just be useful as a start-up way to have a restroom until you are completely building a more permanent one. If your properties are particularly large, you might find that putting in an outhouse at the far end will be helpful when walking around so that you don't have to hike all the way back to your home for number two.

Composting Toilet

This isn't very attractive for everyone but it's actually really great. A composting toilet does not use water. If you remember from the earlier chapter on setting up your water, toilet flushes account for a huge amount of the water that you go through.

Composting toilets can be purchased or built from scratch. You won't need a septic system, so long as you have a good means of disposing of your gray water.

Essentially, this is a system to dump in a bucket and turn your own waste into human compost. Yes, that sounds pretty gross, but it's not as bad as you think. You save a lot of water, and it's very eco-friendly.

Your waste is caught into a bucket with sawdust. The sawdust works a lot like cat litter, it absorbs your waste and also cuts down on the smell. The drier, the better. Some have two separate chambers: one for urine and one for feces.

In your home, you're going to want a fan system to ventilate odors out of your home. Some water mixed with vinegar in a spray bottle can also help a lot.

When you've got a full bucket, haul it out to your composting heap. This is by far the greenest option of all of them. If you are particularly concerned about conservation, this is your best bet.

One way to know who your real friends are is to invite them for a soak in a hot tub hooked up to a compost heat system, heated using your own human manure.

An Outline to Start Your New Home

This is the order of operations to get your homestead off the ground. You can use this as a general outline or like a worksheet, a place to get your mind moving and to get the process of planning moving.

Step One: Make a Decision

This is the biggest step of all. Simply choose if you want to do it. You will need to consider if this is good for your family overall. Make sure that everyone involved understands and is happy to participate. If you have a spouse and children, they need to be okay with all this stuff, too.

Step Two: Planning

The more planning you do, the easier and smoother all the rest of the steps are.

- Figure out your budget.

- Research locations.

- Choose a state and county.

- If you are moving far away, you will have to figure out work if you can't do it remotely—that might mean looking for a new job.

- Calculate your power consumption; estimate how much power you can generate.

- Calculate your water consumption; estimate how much water you can produce.

You want to have an estimate of all the material costs. If there's going to be an interruption to your income, that's going to have to be figured out. There's the price of land and if you live in a state with property taxes.

You also want a buffer room. It is a sure thing that things will go wrong. That's not an off-grid thing, that's a life thing. You might make an error and wire up your electrical system wrong and accidentally torch your inverter. You might have horrendous weather that slows you down. Maybe a clever fox finds their way into your chicken coop. Things always go wrong, and they take time, energy, and money to make them right.

Step Three: Find Land

Once all the other considerations have been weighed, and you know what you are looking for, go find it and buy it.

The two most important things are:

- a place where you are actually allowed to live off-grid without too much interference from red tape and regulation.

- a source of water.

If you are going to need a deep well, get that scheduled and have them come to do that early. If they can't find water, and there is no other good source, this spot is a bust. There's no reason to sink more money or energy into it. Provided that goes well (no pun intended), carry on!

If you don't have a mailbox, you are going to want to get a P.O. box so that you can receive mail and packages.

Step Four: Make a Shelter

Move to your new place. You're going to need a place to sleep. It's fine to start with something small like a camper, a trailer, or even a van if you can stand it. It's definitely recommended that you start in the spring when the temperature is just starting to warm up, and you have more warm months to get started.

If you have a family, they don't all have to come at this point. They can hang back while you get things prepared. It might require some trips back and forth; it might be a process.

Step Four can stay with the temporary place or you can build a more permanent system as you go along. Step Four also fits between every other step.

Step Five: Get Your Baseline

You have a temporary shelter. You also need electricity, water, and food.

Get yourself a gas-powered generator. This is a temporary power source, just until you can get your sustainable system operational.

You need water. You can have it delivered or you can haul it yourself.

Food will be the same grocery-bought stuff you always use.

You'll also need a place to relieve yourself. If you have a trailer or a camper, that's covered. If not, you will need a bucket full of sawdust or an outhouse for the time being.

Garbage can be put in a can or bags and taken to the dump as needed.

You need to get some kind of communication system up as quickly as possible. Depending on how far out your new home is, you may not be able to catch a signal. You can buy a signal booster and attach it to a small tower. That can give you a lot more range. If that doesn't do the trick, consider getting a satellite Internet service.

You're going to want to be able to call for help in an emergency, check the weather, and look up how-to guides when you run into things you don't know how to do. Communication is mandatory.

You now have your baseline. You have all the basic needs covered. As this project continues, each one of those will be replaced with a sustainable system.

Step Six: Electricity

Set up your electrical system. You need your solar panels and/or wind turbines up. You need to get them hooked up safely.

You need a location to house the power system. That probably means building a shed to house everything away from the elements, especially water. Run your connections from your power source. Hook up your AC inverter, batteries, charge controller, fuses, bus bars, etc. Get that all wired up. Contact an electrician if you need to. Safety first!

Step Seven: Water

Now that you have power, you can operate pumps. Once you can have operational pumps, you can get water. Your next task is to hook up to your water source. If you have tanks/cisterns, pipes, and filters ready to go, you are in business. If you have a house built, that means hooking that up. Life just got a lot easier. Also, you can now heat your water, which is a big deal if you've been living without it for a little while.

Step Eight: Waste

Now that you have water, you can hook that up to a septic system. Congratulations if you were using a bucket before because you can now use a toilet!

Step Nine: Start Your Farm

Now that you have working water, you can start your farm and your composting.

Set up a garden and/or build a greenhouse, and get started on any planting.

If you are keeping animals, build them a coop, barn, fenced-in area, or whatever they need.

You are really rolling now!

Step Ten: Do Whatever You Want

You should have all the basic ingredients for self-sustenance: shelter, electricity, water, and food. You can use a toilet and take a shower.

These may not be completely up and running quite yet—you may have hiccups. If necessary, there's no shame in supplementing yourself with visits to the store if you need to.

Where you go from here is entirely up to you. You may find that you want to start upgrading some new systems. You may find that one of the systems you've already built can be built better or optimized.

All the necessities are taken care of. What you do next is whatever you want to do!

Conclusion

Now that we're at the end of the book, you may have started working out a rough sketch of the home you want to build. Maybe you've got your ideal state narrowed down to a few. You've got some ideas about what your home will look like, how you think you can power it, and how to supply water into it.

That's good—get that rough sketch, but don't try to put the ink down on this paper in your imagination just yet. Once you get started, there are going to be a lot of changes and adaptations that you will make along the way. Don't get too hung up on a perfect and idealized version of your homestead. Instead, you and the land should meet each other halfway and figure it out together.

This one book is not going to be nearly enough to teach you everything that you should or want to know. There is a lot more to raising chickens and growing tomatoes than we could possibly cover in these few pages. One of the most important things you should do is continue learning.

When you decide you want to set up your own AC converter, but you don't know the first thing about electricity, you're going to have to read another book about that. Just absorb as much as you can. There are so many other homesteaders and off-grid people out there. There are many forums full of people that are eager to talk to you and share tips. There are countless websites full of great information that can teach you a lot and point you in the right direction.

We know that you're curious about moving off-grid, but at this stage, you're probably more than curious. If you didn't like the idea or didn't sound like it was for you, you probably would have stopped reading this book halfway through earlier, but because you read it from the front to the back, you're still interested.

If you are so interested and have the means and opportunity, We would definitely recommend that you take this on. This is not something we would encourage a half-interested person to do, but if you have made it to the conclusion of this book, you are feeling excited, and you are thinking about all the different projects that you could do and only things you want to learn, then we say follow that instinct. Take it to its ultimate conclusion. Find your own independence, self-reliance, and environmental consideration, and build yourself a place that you will be happy and free.

One Last Thing

We spend so much of our modern lives making things that only exist virtually. Many of us spend a third of our day operating computers. Money people collate tables and leverage financial instruments to make money. Software engineers write complex algebraic formulas to develop a cell phone app. Marketing people look at charts and figures that tell them what people want, without ever talking to people.

So much of what we do isn't material. It exists as an abstraction. People are aching to do something real, tangible, and right here. You'll see it in little ways.

You see people taking on knitting as a hobby, which was formerly considered something that old women do, but young women have suddenly taken an interest in crocheting and other crafts—things that require physical contact.

People are suddenly taking up hobbies like ax throwing and bowhunting.

People get on the Internet and look at videos of people building furniture from scratch.

People start brewing their own beer at home.

People seem to be yearning for another era where people worked with their hands, and when they were done working, there was something tangible in front of them— something that they could be proud of. Instead of working a job and seeing numbers appear in a bank account so they can purchase objects made on the other side of the world, they just want to make something themselves and have it. They want to see the fruits of their own labor and hold on to it like a trophy or a memento—some kind of physical reminder that they can be proud of.

You can feel it too, can't you? Building a life off-grid is not weird. What's weird is living in tiny concrete boxes, stacked hundreds of feet tall, in a gray, concrete place where every day, you see thousands of people walk past you, and you don't know a single one of them.

If you want to try something new—if you want to craft the environment into a place just for you—then you are like many others. Many of them are less smart and talented than you are. If they can do it, you can, too.

References

Average Annual Precipitation for Missouri. (n.d.).
    Current Results.
    https://www.currentresults.com/Weather/Miss
    ouri/average-yearly-precipitation.php

Buri, R. (2017). Solar-roof-solar-energy. In *pixabay.com*.
    https://cdn.pixabay.com/photo/2017/08/21/20
    /29/solar-2666770_960_720.jpg

Cloud, B. (2018). Lake in forest. In *unsplash.com*.
    https://images.unsplash.com/photo-
    1542849922-a7e0aeb0ff84?ixlib=rb-
    1.2.1&ixid=MnwxMjA3fDB8MHxwaG90by1wY
    WdlfHx8fGVufDB8fHx8&auto=format&fit=crop
    &w=1534&q=80

Dais, W. (2011). chicken-coop-farm-chickens-coop. In
    pixabay.com.
    https://cdn.pixabay.com/photo/2014/05/14/08
    /02/chicken-coop-343942_960_720.jpg

Ellis, K. (2018). Triangle house. In *unsplash.com*.
    https://images.unsplash.com/photo-
    1525113990976-
    399835c43838?ixid=MnwxMjA3fDB8MHxwaG9
    0by1wYWdlfHx8fGVufDB8fHx8&ixlib=rb-
    1.2.1&auto=format&fit=crop&w=700&q=80

Giannatti, D. (2019). Outhouse door. In *unsplash.com*.
    https://images.unsplash.com/photo-
    1548097751-
    193b78ef6823?ixid=MnwxMjA3fDB8MHxwaG9
    0by1wYWdlfHx8fGVufDB8fHx8&ixlib=rb-
    1.2.1&auto=format&fit=crop&w=639&q=80

Glenn, K. (2018). Green dome near brown wooden
    dock. In *unsplash.com*.
    https://images.unsplash.com/photo-
    1521401830884-6c03c1c87ebb?ixlib=rb-
    1.2.1&ixid=MnwxMjA3fDB8MHxwaG90by1wY
    WdlfHx8fGVufDB8fHx8&auto=format&fit=crop
    &w=1500&q=80

Gomez, J. (2019). Wood stove. In *unsplash.com*.
    https://images.unsplash.com/photo-
    1564848534637-f57f9b1eb36e?ixlib=rb-
    1.2.1&ixid=MnwxMjA3fDB8MHxwaG90by1wY
    WdlfHx8fGVufDB8fHx8&auto=format&fit=crop
    &w=632&q=80

Gruebner, O., Rapp, M. A., Adli, M., Kluge, U., Galea, S.,
    & Heinz, A. (2017). Cities and Mental Health.
    Deutsches Arzteblatt international, *114*(8), 121–
    127. https://doi.org/10.3238/arztebl.2017.0121

How We Use Water. (n.d.). United States Environmental
    Protection Agency (EPA).
    https://www.epa.gov/watersense/how-we-use-
    water

Jesus, J. (n.d.). Photo-of-man-standing-surrounded-by-green-leaf-plants. In *pexels.com*. https://images.pexels.com/photos/1084540/pexels-photo-1084540.jpeg?auto=compress&cs=tinysrgb&dpr=2&h=650&w=940

Lechner, G. (2020). Black and white wooden house. In *unsplash.com*. https://images.unsplash.com/photo-1580856942656-d4416b6e5c2e?ixlib=rb-1.2.1&ixid=MnwxMjA3fDB8MHxwaG90by1wYWdlfHx8fGVufDB8fHx8&auto=format&fit=crop&w=1563&q=80

Living, O. G. (2020, February 26). *How to go off grid for $10k or less*. Off Grid Living. https://offgridliving.net/go-off-grid-10k/

PublicDomainPictures. (2010). Clean-countryside-drink-garden. In *pixabay.com*. https://cdn.pixabay.com/photo/2012/03/03/22/59/clean-21479_960_720.jpg

Timmer, K. (2019). Brown wood house. In *unsplash.com*. https://images.unsplash.com/photo-1568659585069-facb248c4935?ixlib=rb-1.2.1&ixid=MnwxMjA3fDB8MHxwaG90by1wYWdlfHx8fGVufDB8fHx8&auto=format&fit=crop&w=1500&q=80

www.ingramcontent.com/pod-product-compliance
Lightning Source LLC
Chambersburg PA
CBHW060042100426
42742CB00014B/2674